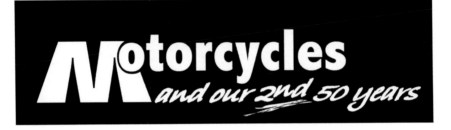

Reg Kittrelle

An Owner's Manual
for Riders over 50

Excuse me...

Reg Kittrelle
reg.kittrelle@comcast.net

Printed in the United States of America
   by Mira Digital Publishing
   www.mirabooksmart.com
First Printing, July 2015
Second Printing, October 2015
Third Printing, November 2015
Fourth Printing, January 2016
Fifth Printing, October 2016
Sixth Printing, January 2017

Published by

ISBN 978-0-9861 1590-0-8

Design and layout by author
© Reg Kittrelle January 2016

It is a bit egocentric to have listed myself as the author. Yeah, I tapped out all words, but if the truth be known, were I left to my own devices the result would have been a mess.

I needed help in any number of areas to get around my ignorance, procrastination, and mulishness. Fortunately I was able to draw from a remarkable well of friends with the talents I lacked. If you like what you read, you can thank them. If you don't like what you read it's probably because I didn't listen to them.

Special Thanks

Lora Sutherland
As my life's primary copy editor, my wife has saved me from embarrassment on any number of occasions, and certainly that held true here. But most of all, I owe her Big Time for the patience she's shown with this effort.

Chelsea Adams, Editor
At one point I accused Chelsea, my editor, of having "savaged" my writing. I can now say that I am so fortunate that she did just that. Great editor, great person.

Birgit Heidgen, Graphic Artist
I naively thought that designing and laying out this book would be something I could knock out quickly. What happened quickly is that I was in over my head. Without Birgit's help you might as well be reading this on the back of a paper towel.

Aaron Bishop, Certified Physical Trainer
Never has one man caused me so much pain ...and I can't thank him enough for setting me on the right path towards physical fitness. (I'm working at it, Aaron, I'm working!)

Rebecca Hazelton, Functional Nutritionist and Physical Trainer
For helping me to recognize that not everything we're putting in our mouths qualifies as food. www.choosinghealthnow.com

Michael Troutman, DMG Images
Lensman Michael did everything he could to make a 72-year-old man look decent enough while exercising. A remarkable photographer. wwwdmgimages.com

Carla King, Adventurer, Author, Entrepreneur
Many thanks to Carla for pointing me in the right directions. If you need this kind of help you can find her at www.SelfPubBootCamp.com

Website?

www.MotorcyclesAnd2nd50.com

Throughout this book I cite numerous references for the information presented, and mention a number of different products.

You can find more information on both on our website under the "Resources" button at the top of the page.

And, of course, the T-shirt is available on our website.

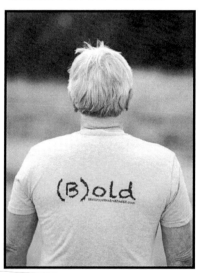

About the author...

Note: As the author's photo is shown more than enough times throughout this book we thought you would rather see a nice picture of banana bread. Besides, everyone likes banana bread whereas with the author it could go either way.

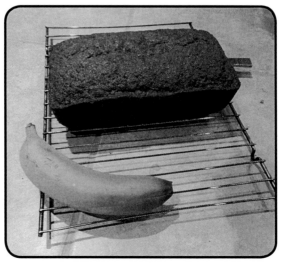

Reg Kittrelle

Starting with a couple of brief rides on a Jawa Perak 250 in the early 1950s Reg's obsession with motorcycles has let his wallet drag him onto 60-plus motorcycles, the starting grid of dirt track and roadraces, a parts and accessories business, a dirt bike dealership, various industry PR jobs, a publishing business (*Thunder Press, Battle2win Magazine*), motorcycle event promotion, and a wealth of memories, some of which he actually believes.

Inside

 ONE

Who We Are

We are the people we never thought we'd become: old. Is that a bad thing? Nope!

 TWO

Do Something About It

Either you do something about it, or it will do something about you. Trust me, you won't like the second option.

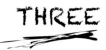 **THREE**

As We Eat So We Ride

"Eat to ride, ride to eat."
You might just be doing that wrong.

FOUR

The Other Part of Fitness

Making sure that everything we
need is as fit as it should be

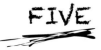

FIVE

Hardware

The "bolts" that go along with us "nuts"

SIX

This Time It's Personal

Just you and me

Before You Start...

If a book can have an attitude then this one's can be found in a poem by Welsh poet Dylan Thomas: *Do Not Gentle Go Into That Good Night.*

Do not go gentle into that good night,
Old age should burn and rave at close of day;
Rage, rage against the dying of the light.

If you're a motorcycle rider over the age of 50 you are a member of the largest and fastest growing segment of the riding population. You are also among the most ignored, as the 18 to 35 demographic get most of the marketing and industry attention. That's OK though, by our age we've come to realize that youth *thinks* it rules.

But what about us older riders? Our needs and concerns are slightly different (and sometimes a lot more than slightly) from those of younger riders. Addressing these is what this book is all about; it's about examining the differences between the rider we are now and the rider we used to be, and learning how to deal with those differences so we can keep riding regardless of our age.

We're special, us old dogs. We're special because we've managed to survive the road, increase our skills, and bank a ton of memories that only time and experience can accrue. But we have also changed over the years. If you're at all like me, you've put on a few pounds, have a persistent ache or pain that's become a constant companion, and your riding habits are possibly changing from long hauls to shorter, less challenging trips. Maybe some of these changes have started you thinking that your riding days are nearing an end.

Stop right there. Your aches and pains are real, but that doesn't mean your saddle days are numbered. In fact, chances are the opposite is true. This book has two purposes: to build awareness of the physical and mental factors of old age, and what you can do about them, and to show that your riding days — regardless of your age — are not necessarily nearing an end. Despite your age, if you are in reasonable physical condition, your best riding days could be in your future. I'll show you the steps to take to assure that riding a motorcycle in your 50s, 60s, 70's, and even beyond that can be some of the most enjoyable times you've had.

and...

1) I use the pronouns "he" and "him" throughout this book. This is not to imply any bias, or to exclude women riders but, rather, for simplicity's sake; writing "he or she," or "him or her" gets clunky and is just awkward writing to me. However I do believe that most of what you'll read here applies to both men and women.

2) I've omitted discussing off-road motorcycles other than in passing. I have very special memories of years of off-road riding, and highly recommend that everyone try it, but given that the dirt end of the riding spectrum is primarily (although not exclusively!) the domain of young riders, I have omitted that segment of our sport.

3) Several of the subjects I cover in this book involve mention of the "newest" technology, which means that by the time you read this what's "new" will likely have changed. Change doesn't invalidate what I've written; think of these lessons as a foundation on which to better understand the latest and greatest, whatever that passing trend may currently be.

4) Since I tend to wander a bit with the subjects I've chosen to write about, I've structured each chapter in this book to be freestanding. That is, you can skip about the book without losing anything.

5) This is really important:

This is not a book of medical cures, or wonder diets, and it won't help you get perfect abs in 30 days. I am an experienced rider, but I am not a doctor, physical trainer, therapist, or dietician. While the information I offer is based on solid science, I'm sure you're smart enough to know that this information should be considered general in nature, as each of us can react differently to given situations. Consider what you find here to be opinion, then do three things: think about it, weigh the pros and cons, then, before you embark on any program of exercise or change your diet, I strongly recommend that you consult your doctor.

Got that?

A note to all you layout artists:

In addition to writing this book, I thought it would be fun to also lay it out. I quickly learned that my definition of "fun" might need a bit of adjustment. The application I used was InDesign CS5.

I'm writing this note after reviewing the final proof from the printer. Despite numerous reviews and edits, I've discovered a handful of small layout errors. Errors that I am not able to change due to time constraints. I'd appreciate it if you would never speak of these errors.

Thank you,

ONE

50

60

who we are...

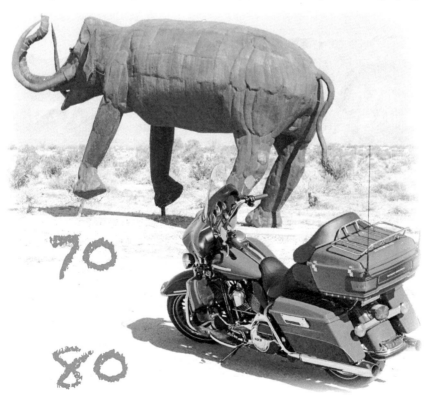

70

80

1.

*Every rider starts with a bag full of luck and
an empty bag of experience. The trick is to fill
one before the other runs out.*

Anon.

Why this book?

My riding was getting sloppy. In particular, I was having some
balance problems with low-speed turns and my lines in fast
sweepers had developed a tendency to wander a bit. Initially, this didn't
particularly bother me as I'd been riding less than usual. My thought
was, "OK, I just need to spend a bit more time in the saddle."

I live in the Santa Cruz mountains of northern California. Tight,
winding motorcycle roads that place a premium on proper wheel placement surround my home. I've always thought of these roads as my
private training ground, and I access them by merely going to the end of
my driveway. It was time to put a wheel to my "training ground" once
again. I spent the best part of a day chasing apexes, but it didn't help
much. Yes, I knocked off some rough edges, but I still felt I'd lost a step.

I've never been a motorcycle hero. Competent, yes, but you'd not
mistake me for a two-wheeled star. I've raced dirt track and roadraced
enough to understand the sports, and with just enough success to feel
good about it, but not enough to brag. Still, I've prided myself on my
street skills, and now they seemed to be eroding.

I had a fleeting thought that, at 72 years of age, maybe I ought to
thank the two-wheeled gods for the long riding career I've had and just
hang up the helmet. Note that I said "fleeting" because that thought was
quickly pushed aside by the next one, "uh... no." My life, my friends,
my business... they all revolve around riding a motorcycle. Like it or
not, the majority of my life has been defined by motorcycles, and I
wasn't — and am not — ready to release the D-ring for the last time.
Not yet. That unsettling thought caused me to recall the many competent
riders I knew in their 70's — and older — and that the number of

50-plus riders was very large indeed. Surely, I reasoned, I was not the only one to have reached this riding crisis point.

Next, a bit of research followed and the more I delved into the subject of age and riding motorcycles, the more I was convinced I wasn't yet at the end of my riding road. "Live to ride, ride to live" is an over-used phrase found on any number of T-shirts, vests, and needled biceps throughout the world of motorcycles. You've heard it, certainly, but have you ever thought about what it means or, more correctly, what it means to you? For me — at 72 — it means understanding what I am up against as an older rider and, most importantly, what I can do about it. In other words, learning to live in a way that keeps me riding, and to ride in a way that keeps me living.

I wasn't ready to give up the saddle, despite my getting older, so instead of posting my Triumph on craigslist I began writing this book. For me, this book is all about truly learning to live right so that I can ride right. I hope the research and my thoughts within these pages helps to extend the life in your riding, and the riding in your life.

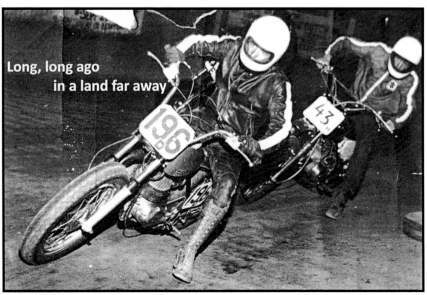

Long, long ago in a land far away

Hayward Speedway 1968.
Bultaco Pursang 250. I'm wearing one of the original Bell "Star" helmets, Langlitz Leathers and, of course, lineman's boots. Those of you who raced dirt track during this era will recognize this picture as one from the talented camera of Bill Spencer.

2.

Age vs. Old

If you're 25 years old and an Olympic gymnast, you're old. If you're 35 and a MotoGP racer, you're old. If you're 40 and an NFL lineman, you're old. Proof of this is as close as the sports pages of your daily paper. Youth indeed may be fleeting, but that's ridiculous.

However true it might be from an ultimate physical peak stand-point, the good news is those examples have little relevance to the majority of us; we're not gymnasts, GP racers, or linebackers. The bad news, on the other hand, is that while professional sports may be a bit of an unreal world to us mortals, we are influenced — unfortunately — by its idea of "old." Couple this with our youth-obsessed culture and it's no wonder that the fear of growing old ranks right up at the top of everyone's "Not looking forward to it" list.

What we have lost in all these "how old is old" comparisons is not our fleeting youth, but our perspective. That we are continually aging is an indisputable fact — deal with it. As to whether or not we are old, well, that depends upon your point of view. Depressed by that sports page reference? Try this instead; if you're 55 and a Supreme Court justice, you're young. In this light, it's obvious that while age is an objective evaluation, old is open to discussion, and is very much a subjective evaluation. Furthermore, being old is largely a decision. That is, regardless of how many birthday cakes you've tasted, you can decide not to be "old," except on your terms.

The Stages of Life

Medical science generally agrees on various stages of life and ties them directly back to age. Typically, if you are between 20 and 35 you are considered a young adult. From 35 to 45 you are thought of as young middle-aged, followed by later middle-age from 45 to 65. Old age is broken into three stages; early old from 65 to 75, middle old takes up the

75 to 85 period, and very old kicks in at 85. The problem with information like this is that it slices and slots us into categories that may not be reflective of the way we actually live. Does it make sense, for example, to group a healthy, active 60-year-old motorcycle rider in with a 40-year-old couch spud whose exercise is limited to popping a top and pushing a remote button? One of these people is definitely old, the other not necessarily so.

Different Measurements of Age

To me, there are actually five different age measurements: chronologic, genetic, social, mirror, and marketing.

Our **chronologic age** is an absolute; it is measured by the calendar, and is not open to dispute (unless you're an aging Hollywood star). Though obviously relevant, it is certainly not the deciding factor that determines whether we are "getting old," or are "too old" to ride.

Genetic age is determined by inherited traits. Our gender, hair color, body shape and size (called a *somatype*), disposition towards certain diseases, and the thousands of other unique features that make us the individuals that we are, are all hardwired within our genetic structure – our DNA. This is the physical hand that we are dealt but, if we play our cards right, we can have a significant impact on our genetic age.

What we have lost in all these "how old is old" comparisons is not our fleeting youth, but our perspective.

The third measurement is our **social age**. This is largely influenced by social norms and customs. In other words, the expectations that others — and ourselves — impose upon us that influence how old we act and feel. Illustrating this are the examples at the beginning of this chapter. In the world of most professional sports, once you've hit 30 years old people start wondering when you're going to stop playing and get a real job. Forty years of age? Whoa ... all that's left is for the genetically disposed very large woman to start singing. You're old, you're finished. Yet, in the world of business and politics it's often thought that you don't really hit your peak until you're in your forties or fifties. In that social world you're not old; you're just hitting your stride.

5

Our social age can be improved by largely ignoring the subtle pressure that comes from the organizations and people that surround us. Those of us in my age group (70's) experience this on a somewhat continual basis. Usually it pops up with the well-meant question, "So, what are you doing in your retirement?" The social norm dictates that we can't be anything but retired.

Our **mirror age** reflects the physical progression, or digression, of our bodies; the loss of muscle mass, reduced lung capacity, and reduced bone density that we all eventually experience. In many ways this age measurement contains the most controllable variables as it is influenced by our choice of lifestyle. For example, while we can do nothing about our genetic makeup we can control habits to mitigate our genetic disposition and, thus, our mirror age. If, for example, our *somatotype* is that of an *endomorph* we will be inclined to be large-boned, wide of hip, and overweight. While those characteristics are an integral part of our DNA, we can influence them somewhat through diet and exercise.

And then there's our **marketing age**. This can be the most insidious aging factor because it is primarily about money, and we are virtually encased by marketing. In his 1997 book Data Smog, journalist David Shenk wrote that, "In 1971 the average American was targeted by at least 560 daily advertising messages. Twenty years later, that number had risen sixfold, to 3,000 messages a day." When you consider that this datum is more than two decades old, then add in the exponential growth of the Internet since then —and our interaction with it— the word pervasive only begins to describe the impact that advertising has on us. I need to add, these are controversial numbers, as you can find experts who argue them both higher and lower. Regardless of the exact number, it's irrefutable that we are being inundated with advertising on a continual basis.

Our Different Ages

Chronologic
According to the calendar
Genetic
Thanks, Mom & Dad
Social
What *others* see
Mirror
What *we* see
Marketing
What commerce sees

It's Up to You to Decide How Old You Are

Now consider the content of this advertising. It is largely focused on the benefits of being young and — if you're not — showing you how to recapture your youth, or at least a semblance of it. When old age is shown it is usually as a negative counterpoint, as in a "before" picture. Our marketing age has, in many ways, the most impact on whether or not we are considered old, or feel old. Our culture — and a large part of the rest of the world — covets youth. Product marketeers work hard to attract that prime demographic, the Holy Grail that is the 18- to 34-year-olds. They do this not because this group is in its peak earning years — that would be the 45 to 55 age group — but because marketers know if they capture a young mind with their product that person will likely stay with it a long time. Whereas the wealthier but older groups, well, they're gonna die off sooner.

Marketing ...can have a tendency to marginalize anyone who is not in the younger half of life.

One of the depressing side effects of this marketing —and the attendant social pressures— is that it can have a tendency to marginalize anyone who is not in the younger half of life. In other words, if we're not "young," then we must be "old," and suffer all the bad stuff that comes with it. All of which can grind against our self-image and self-esteem. If it is continually implied through marketing that we are "old," well then, we must be. Right?

Or not. While we can do nothing about our chronologic and genetic ages — that's a hard, carved-in-stone number — we *can* make the choice as to whether or not we want to live by a definition pressed on us by others, or create our own proud, physically fit definition.

3.

Two old riders had been friends for many decades,
having shared all kinds of activities and adventures.
Stopping for coffee during a recent ride, one rider
stared at the the other and said,
>   *"Now don't get mad at me.*
>   *I know we've been friends for a long time,*
>   *but I just can't think of your name!*
>   *I've thought and thought, but I just can't*
>   *remember it. Could you tell me what it is?"*
His friend glared at him. For at least two minutes
he just stared and glared, and finally said,
>   *"uh... how soon do you need to know?"*

                                                    Anon.

Who is Old?

According to the Motorcycle Industry Council (MIC) in 2008 there were 11,099,615 motorcycles owned in the U.S. Skip ahead to 2012 and that number dropped to 10,319,500 motorcycles owned, reflecting the effect of the serious market loss we experienced during the four-year gap between the two measurements.

Motorcycling is usually thought of as a young person's sport. Yet, look at the chart that follows and you'll see that the largest group of motorcycle owners slot into that "50 and up" category. It's also notable that this group increased by nine percent in 2012 over the 2008 number. I'm not a fan of euphemisms (I find, for example, "young at heart" and "70 years young" more than a bit patronizing) so throughout this book I'm going to refer to us —this 50 and up group— as "old," or "older" riders. I realize that this term might not sit well with everyone, but I think that's because "old" has been co-opted by The Young Side. It has become a synonym for obsolete, or useless, rather than what *Webster's Dictionary* intended with its respectful, "of long standing" definition. I take pride in being called an old rider; it has a nice, respectful ring to it. The focus of this book begins just about where the chart leaves off; the aged "50 and up" rider.

Age Distribution of Riders

	PERCENTAGE	
Age	2008	2012
Under 18	4	2
18-24	11	10
25-29	8	9
30-34	9	11
35-39	10	8
40-49	28	21
50 and up	29	38

There's something about that half-century mark that sends a shiver down the spines of most, motorcycle rider or not. Around that age you begin to realize that Boy Wonder is dead, your path in life has probably been set, and the definition of mortality looms ever larger. This is the age when your doctor starts campaigning for all manner of invasive tests, AARP begins its assault on your mailbox, and little things like losing your keys causes great concern amongst your loved ones. And possibly the worst part of this milestone —millstone is more correct— is that friend and foe alike will not let you forget it; birthday presents generally have "Over The Hill" writ large, and adult diaper jokes start to appear all too often.

There is a subset of this 50 and up group that the MIC data does not address: experience. A 55-year-old on a motorcycle does not necessarily mean that he has a similarly long history in the saddle. In fact, there's enough anecdotal evidence out there to make me believe that a significantly large percentage of chronologically older riders do not fit the "long-standing" definition. They may have the years under their belts, but not the miles.

I would hope that, regardless of your age, you begin viewing the term "old" in its rightful context, and that you make the decision of just how old you want to be and not let it be the decision of others.

4.

*70-year-old George went for his annual physical.
He told the doctor that he felt fine, but often had to
go to the bathroom during the night. Then he said,
"But you know Doc, I'm blessed. God knows my
eyesight is going, so he puts on the light when I pee,
and turns it off when I'm done!"*

*Later in the day the doctor called George's wife and
said, "Your husband's test results were fine, but he
said something strange that has been bugging me.
He claims that God turns the light on and off for
him when he uses the bathroom at night."*

*Thelma exclaimed, "That old fool! He's been peeing
in the refrigerator again!"*

Anon.

What Age Does to Our Bodies

There's no masking it, this part of the book is filled with bad news you don't necessarily want to hear. Some of it is age-related bad news, some of it is lifestyle-related bad news, all of it is moderately depressing bad news. Unless, that is, you shift your mindset.

Contrary to what you may be feeling right now, I did not write this chapter to depress the hell out of you. Rather, this chapter — and every one before and after it — was created to help you. Sure, this isn't the lightest chapter in the book, but it does end on a light note. See, every one of the "downhill" conditions covered in this chapter can be improved upon with a few small lifestyle changes — but you can't fix anything until you recognize something may be broken.

This chapter is all about understanding your condition so you don't have to fall victim to it. In other words, shifting your mindset from feeling sorry for yourself to taking charge of yourself.

First Things First: The Truth Is... We're Dying

Back in 1998 an alternative rock band, Cake, released the song "Sheep Go to Heaven." It's a depressing four minutes of music ideally suited to be played as one takes a swan dive off a tall building. I mention it because it contains a line somewhat appropriate to our subject:

"As soon as you're born, you start dying..."

There's a lot of truth to that if, for no other reason, the countdown clock starts ticking as soon as you take your first breath. That said, for most panic doesn't kick in until we start to physically see and feel signs of aging; that point when we look in the mirror and see someone that more closely resembles our parents than it does us. Experts are a little vague as to when we start losing it — hair, muscle, height, eyesight, et al— but most cite "middle age" as the turning point. That means somewhere around 45-ish years of age (and this can vary widely) things start to literally and metaphorically go downhill. Fortunately we don't need to run through the complete itinerary of aging effects here, but we do need to look at those that have the most significant impact on our ability to ride a motorcycle. As depressing as all this might sound, try to keep something in mind as you continue through this chapter: every one of the conditions listed can be improved upon. Also remember that not making a choice is making a choice. If you read this chapter then choose to sit back and let these things happen to you, remember, it was your choice to do so.

10 Conditions That Can Impact Older Riders

Brittle Bones

For both men and women the mass and density — and thus, the strength — of our bones peak out in our 20's or 30's. After those decades the bone-building process usually begins to reverse itself, with the effect being that our skeleton becomes smaller, and our bones thinner and less dense. This happens because as we age our bodies do not replace broken-down bone matter (a normal process) as quickly as when we were young. As you can imagine, having weak and brittle bones is not a condition that works well with motorcycle riding and, in particular, motorcycle falling. Medically, low bone mass is known as *osteopenia*, with the continual thinning of the bones leading to *osteoporosis*. Technically, it is not the density of our bones that is affected but, rather, our bone mineral density (BMD). This refers to the amount of calcium and other strengthening mineral matter in the bones, a source of a bone's strength — in particular, calcium. Simply put, the lower the BMD, the more prone a bone is to fracture.

There are a couple of prevalent misconceptions surrounding osteoporosis. First off, osteoporosis is not necessarily an inevitability of aging. It is a disease, but one that many experts claim to be not only curable but also preventable and reversible. In addition to age, there are also controllable contributing factors that negatively influence BMD. In particular, factors like obesity, excessive alcohol consumption, smoking, and a sedentary lifestyle have all been shown to weaken bones. It's important to note that all of those factors result from decisions we make. Yes, there can be a genetic element to osteoporosis, but even if you get the osteoporosis gene you still have lifestyle options that can improve bone mineral density.

...though osteoporosis is approximately four times more prevalent with women than with men, it is not exclusive to women.

Secondly, though osteoporosis is approximately four times more prevalent with women than with men, it is not exclusive to women. There are several reasons why women are more prone to osteoporosis than men, including a generally smaller skeletal size and postmenopausal effects that tend to cause rapid loss of bone density. However, once men reach their mid-60's they are on par with women as far as the rate of bone density loss is concerned.

According to the Center for Disease Control, falling down is continually the leading cause of injury death among people 65 or older. This happens for two reasons: first, most in the 65-plus age group have become victims of brittle, easily broken bones, and, second, weakened bones do not heal properly, if at all. Now, considering that most of these elderly broken bones happen in the home at walking speeds or less, you quickly understand how serious throwing yourself off your motorcycle can become, even if you're moving very slowly.

and this... BMD Testing

As older riders it is important that we assess our risk of bone fractures. There are several tests that doctors can perform to measure the density of the minerals in bones, the determining factor of bone strength. Currently, the most widely used is the dual-energy X-ray absorptiometry test, or DXA for short. This test is believed to be the most accurate method of determining your risk of osteoporosis. Ultrasound screening is another popular test method, but it cannot measure the density of critical bones such as those in the hip. Some prefer the ultrasound screening to the DXA test because the ultrasound uses sound waves rather than X-rays, but it really should only be considered a starting point. If low bone density is determined, the next step should be the DXA test.

A DXA test will give you a T-Score, and a Z-Score. The T-Score result is a comparison of your BMD to that of a same gender, healthy 30-year-old male/female (depending on your gender), whereas the Z-Score compares your results with those of the same age and gender.

There are a number of factors involved in determining just who should have a BMD test but, in general, women over the age of 65 and men over the age of 70 should be tested. This is a decision that should be discussed with your doctor.

Loss of Muscle Mass

Medical science refers to the loss of muscle mass and function through aging and inactivity as *sarcopenia*. Physical strength, coordination and balance are adversely affected by this condition. Most reports indicate that sarcopenia noticeably begins in our 40's, though I have seen some reference to it starting as young as the mid-20's. Typically, once you reach your 60's, the loss of muscle mass accelerates. Obviously, loss of strength, a decrease in coordination, and impaired balance directly impact a motorcycle rider.

Operating any motor vehicle requires a significant degree of physical coordination, but a motorcycle places a premium on coordination, as the consequences of poor coordination can be dangerous and possibly deadly. On a very basic level, if we lack the necessary leg strength, holding up a large touring motorcycle can become problematic. Several years ago I wrote an article on a popular trike. During the interview with the company owner I asked him for a profile of his customers. Were they experienced riders, non-riders, young, old; just who are the trike riders? "Frankly," he answered, "the majority of our experienced riders are those who feel they can no longer hold up a large motorcycle." He asked that I not attribute that quote to him. In defense of trike riders, while this may have been true when I asked the question, today's trikes (with no small thanks to the Can-Am Spyder) are attracting a younger, more fit, crowd.

When we're in the saddle we have to coordinate front and rear brakes, clutch, and throttle. Additionally, as our bodies are highly vulnerable to the misdeeds of others (not to mention our own) we need to keep 360 degrees of awareness in action. To accomplish this daunting task it is necessary to first evaluate the input we're receiving from our eyes, our ears, the road, the weather, our motorcycle's performance, and traffic. This microsecond evaluation then tells our hands and feet to apply given amounts of pressure on various levers, and to position our bodies accordingly (for instance, lean in, lean out, countersteer, etc.). If all our various muscles – including our brain – function as they should, there's no problem. However, if our strength, coordination, and balance have significantly diminished, well, that can be a problem. For example, missing a shift might just put you in the path of that car you were trying to avoid, or too much rear brake pressure could cause a slide.

...falling down (without the help of a motorcycle) is the leading cause of death due to injury for people 65 or older.

Impaired Balance

As mentioned earlier, those fun people at the Center for Disease Control have determined falling down (without the help of a motorcycle) is the leading cause of death due to injury for people 65 or older. In 2010 this amounted to over 21,000 deaths for older adults suffering injuries from falling. The primary cause of these falls was twofold: lack of physical strength and balance problems. Balance problems can have other causative factors, such as illness and inner ear problems, but the lack of physical strength — in particular our core strength — will largely determine how well we are able to balance ourselves. And if our balance is impaired, it doesn't take a lot of imagination to see how this condition will negatively affect our riding.

One of the surest signs of aging is decreased physical flexibility. Older people — and sometimes not so old people — often walk in a stiff, stilted manner. Barring injury and/or disease, the reason behind this zombie-like walk is easily explained: it is usually due to muscular atrophy. If a muscle is not used regularly it will lose its elasticity and become less effective (atrophy), resulting in a decreased range of motion.

As a rider, there are two noticeable effects of decreased flexibility. First, is the ability to lift your right leg high enough to clear the saddle when you climb aboard your motorcycle and, second, is the inability to turn your head sufficiently to see behind you, as when changing lanes.

Given that most of these ads featured lithe young women in designer spray paint...

Diminished Core Strength

As I mentioned, my riding was getting a little sloppy. In looking for answers to this — I wasn't ready to write it off as "old age" — the term "core strength" kept popping up in my research. I was familiar with the term insomuch as I continually see it in various local fitness ads trying to sell me Pilates classes (Pilates is a very popular fitness routine and fitness is a cottage industry in my town of Santa Cruz). Given that most of these ads featured lithe young women in designer spray paint, I dismissed this as something I would not want to do. But as I researched deeper, I discovered that the "core strength" idea was very applicable to motorcycle riders – and very attainable without Pilates or a spray can. The idea here is that the muscles of your stomach, side, and lower- and mid-back (also known as your "trunk" or your "core" muscles) function as controlling agents for the rest of your body. Regardless of how large or small the movement of any body part, these core muscles are brought into play. The only time this is not the case is when you are laying flat on your back. Given this, it is easy to see the importance of "core strength."

Let me draw an analogy with our motorcycles. Our core muscles are our body's suspension. If our motorcycle's suspension is weak —

springs are shot, oil is low — we cannot precisely place our wheels and our motorcycle can become very difficult to ride. If our body's "suspension" is weak, we cannot precisely control the movement of our arms, legs, and neck.

One of the common complaints from many motorcycle riders is lower back pain from long hours in the saddle. Absent a prior injury, illness, or obesity, this complaint can be directly traced to a lack of core strength. Seemingly, just sitting in the saddle would not appear to tax our muscles. However, something has to hold up and steady the upper half of our body, which constitutes a major portion of our body's weight — and that "something" is our core muscle structure. The core is continually working at keeping us upright. If you need proof of this, simply place your hand on your side and move your trunk around; you'll feel the muscles working. If these muscles are weak, it will allow our upper body to press down on the hips and spine, putting pressure on any of the more than 50 nerves rooted in the spinal column. The result: back pain. If this happens, it could be said — to continue that motorcycle analogy — that our body's suspension is sacked out.

Slowed Thinking

Cognition is a term that covers our ability to acquire knowledge, make decisions, solve problems, and quickly decide if that car is going to make a left turn directly in front of us.

As we age our ability to recognize, retrieve, and analyze information slows. Citing the reasons for this would be a book-long essay in itself. The physiological basis for this degradation includes, among others, a deterioration of the *hippocampus* (this is the part of the brain that determines whether or not we can find our keys, where we parked our bike, etc.) and a decrease in blood flow to the brain. The latter is critical as our brains are fueled by, and depend upon, oxygen- and nutrient-enriched blood. Additional factors include how our brain absorbs nutrients, and how it repairs itself by processing proteins and hormones.

Research shows that both our lifestyle and genetic structure can contribute to impaired cognition. One of the largest contributing factors is hardening of the arteries (atherosclerosis). This condition results in a narrowing of the arteries due to fat (cholesterol) which hardens into plaque, resulting in reduced blood flow to various body organs such as the brain, heart, liver, and eyes. While genetics can contribute to this condition, it is thought by many that lifestyle is the biggest culprit. Specifically, obesity, lack of exercise, and smoking are huge contributing factors.

Reaction Time Increase

The *American Heritage Dictionary* defines reaction time as, "The interval of time between application of a stimulus and detection of a response." I define it as the interval of time between the 2x4 falling from a truck and me saying, "Ooh, that could leave a mark!"

During that exceedingly short interval, a lot goes on within our body. The basic process goes something like this: Our eyes see an image, send an electrical signal (nerve impulse) to our central nervous system (our brain and spinal cord) which then sends an impulse to our muscles. That interval takes around 18 one-hundredths (0.018) of a second. Gifted athletes can beat that, but it's thought to be impossible to get below a reaction time of 0.010 hundredths of a second without having anticipated the stimulus. To this point, however, we still haven't done anything; the muscles have the message, but haven't contracted. Fortunately, our muscles contract very quickly. It takes something around 60 to 80 micro-seconds for this to happen. So what does this mean as regards to avoiding that dropped 2 x 4?

Let's say I'm traveling at 60 miles per hour; that's 88 feet per second. With that reaction time of around 0.018 of a second, this means I've travelled about five feet before my brain tells my body to take eva-sive action. This may not sound like a lot, but consider the times that you barely missed hitting an obstacle, or rear-ending someone who pulled out in front of you. As we age, the various components of our reaction time have a tendency to lengthen, which means a five-foot reaction delay can easily becomes six, seven, or more feet, thereby reducing our margin of safety drastically.

Impaired Eyesight

You can get away with riding a motorcycle if you are in less than great physical condition, or if your cognitive powers aren't what they used to be. But if your eyesight begins to fail, well, your riding career will soon become toast.

According to the National Eye Institute, *Age-Related Macular*

Degeneration (AMD) is a leading cause of vision loss in older adults. The macula, the most light-sensitive portion of our retinas, is located at the rear of our eyes, and provides the sharpness and clarity (visual acuity) necessary to read, operate a motorcycle and, for that matter, work on a motorcycle. When the macula degenerates, it degrades the amount and quality of light information that is sent to the brain. That is, our vision becomes impaired.

Compounding this is the normal shrinkage of the pupils as we age. Pupils control the amount of light that enters our eyes so any reduction in their size serves to reduce the amount of light that reaches the macula — and accordingly, the amount we can see. Additionally, the lens of the eye has a tendency to yellow as we age, and this can adversely impact color differentiation.

All of this gives old eyes a reduced capacity to detect light contrast. Colors, in effect, become muted and are more difficult to discern. (Could this account for some of those hideous green and yellow pants worn by many older golfers?) This condition is particularly acute in dim light, and at night.

Accurate depth perception is critical to the safe operation of a motorcycle, or any motor vehicle. *Stereopsis* is the medical term for the process that allows us to discern and differentiate objects that are at varying distances from us (binocular disparity). As we age this ability degrades. One of the most prevalent reasons for this is a condition known as *anisometropia*. This is where the focusing abilities of each of our eyes (*presbyopia*) differ from each other. For example, one eye might tend towards nearsightedness (*myopia*), while the other is farsighted (*hyperopia*). Studies have shown that this condition can be as much as 10 times more prevalent with those pushing 75 than it is with children.

Generally, the first significant sign of anisometropia is when a rider mentions that they no longer like to ride at night. Couple differing focusing abilities with the reduced capacity to detect contrast and you can understand why depth perception at night can be a serious problem with older riders.

Loss of Hearing

There is a certain inevitability with regard to hearing loss and old age. While statistics vary, most authorities agree that about 35 percent of us 65- to 74-year-olds suffer some hearing loss. At age 75, the percentage nears 50. As with most all ailments, hearing loss can have several causes, but for our purposes the one that we need to consider is *presbycusis*. This results from the hair cells within our inner ear dying or becoming damaged. These cells sense vibrations and create an electrical signal that is sent to the auditory nerve that carries the signal to the brain. Simply, this is the loss we gradually experience as we age. It has numerous causes including heredity, head injuries, high blood pressure, infection, and loud noise.

That last one in particular — loud noise — is especially applicable to riders. Medically known as noise-induced hearing loss (NIHL) it has as a causative factor as the name implies — duh, loud noise. OK, you might ask, "How do we define loud noise?" The definition of loud can range from a librarian getting upset over a mouse fart, to a pain-inducing unmuffled two-stroke motor. While the subjective definition of "loud" can vary greatly, lucky for us sound — and how much sound is too much sound — is actually very easy to quantify scientifically.

...about 35 percent of us 65- to 74-year-olds suffer some hearing loss.

Sound intensity is measured in decibels (dB) with near-silence rated at 0 dB, and normal conversation at around 50 dB to 70 dB. The important thing to know about decibels is that they are logarithmic, rather than linear numbers. On a linear scale, a change between two numbers is based upon addition, e.g., 10 + 10 = 20. On a logarithmic scale, a change between two numbers is based upon multiplication. For example, a conversation heard at 60 dBs is 10 times more intense than one heard at 50 dBs. Many experts agree that any sound above about 90 dB can cause hearing impairment, and that sustained noise above a 95 dB level will, in all likelihood, cause hearing loss.

The Occupational Safety and Health Administration (OSHA) has established permissible levels of noise exposure in the workplace, per day. For example, OSHA says that eight hours is the maximum exposure for a 90 dB sound level. When the level moves to 95 dB, four hours is the maximum exposure time. And in case you are interested, pain begins at sound levels of 125 dB.

For perspective, here are a few typical sound levels:

Electric hand drill	98 dB
Gas-engined lawn mower	107 dB
Loud rock concert	115 dB

For us riders, potentially harmful noise usually comes from two sources: wind and exhaust pipes. Wind noise is insidious in that we're usually not that conscious of it or, rather, we dismiss it as not being harmful. There have been several reports, however, that show wind noise levels can exceed 100 dB. Reread that above paragraph on OSHA's recommended levels and you see where wind noise is a serious problem. Interestingly, research has also shown that at about 35 mph our exhaust noise is no longer a factor as it fades off behind us.

Where exhaust noise is a factor is when you're riding next to it on a trip. On large motorcycles featuring illegally modified exhaust systems, the sound level can easily exceed 100 dB. Modified exhaust systems is a highly charged subject among riders. At one end of the spectrum are those who believe that "loud pipes save lives." The idea being that inattentive motorists will be made aware that a motorcycle is in the area.

It is my strongly held belief that if you need to resort to loud pipes to save your hide, then maybe a course or two in defensive riding might be in order.

I can find no authoritative study supporting this assertion, but there is some anecdotal evidence that, indeed, some have been saved by a loud exhaust system. In opposition to this group are those riders who prefer the quietude offered by unmodified exhaust systems and seriously question the "loud pipes save lives" position.

I find myself solidly aligned with the "quiet" group. In my younger years I raced two-stroke, unmuffled motorcycles that were without a doubt hugely instrumental in my hearing loss. I love the sound that a big twin in particular can make whether burbling around town, or at full chat out on the highway. I do not, however, enjoy the noise on long trips, nor around town where it garners nothing but justified annoyance from most everyone other than prepubescent children. Additionally, if you've ever traveled long miles next to an obnoxiously loud motorcycle, you've probably come away rethinking your position on this subject.

It is my strongly held belief that if you need to resort to loud pipes to save your hide, then maybe a course or two in defensive riding might be in order.

Heat Intolerance

Yet another health concern that can be related to aging is intolerance to hot weather. I write "can be" because a bit of simple research shows that while later middle-aged (45 to 65) men and women are more prone to suffer from heat intolerance, the reasons behind this probably includes a more sedentary lifestyle, medications used, obesity, and the presence of a disease, rather than just the fact they are old. However, it is well documented that the elderly generally experience a reduction of

and this... Huh?

My hearing loss became noticeable about 20 years ago, at around age 50. Currently, the loss is 60% in my left ear, and 40% in my right ear. I have spent thousands of dollars on various hearing aids, none of which have worked as advertised.

My first indication of hearing loss arrived with a bout of tinnitus. In my case, it was a low-level ringing in my ears that would come and go for no apparent reason. For some, it is a constant, loud roaring sound. While it was certainly irritating, I did nothing about it because I was told that there was nothing that could be done. After a couple of years it disappeared, but was replaced by some hearing loss. This was, and is, the result of multiple factors: first, normal aging and, second, noise-induced hearing loss (NIHL). NIHL is an all-inclusive term that covers any loud noise suffered on an ongoing basis. In my case, there are three damaging components to this.

Beginning in the mid-1960s, I dirt-tracked two-stroke motorcycles for several years — mostly Bultacos. As was the habit of the day, I ran without a silencer. This was the heyday of "scrambles" racing, so it wasn't unusual to have a couple of hundred unsilenced motorcycles show up on race days. At the time, the sound was pure music to my ears. That it might be eroding my hearing was never a concern.

...continued

Huh? *continued...*
The second component to my hearing loss occurred in the same time-frame: music. Very loud music. More specifically, music concerts at the Fillmore Auditorium and Avalon Ballroom in San Francisco. The idea then was to get as close to the massive speakers as possible so that Janis Joplin's music literally moved you. Thirdly, and probably the most damaging of the components, was —and is— wind noise from the riding of motorcycles for more than 50 years.

Hearing loss is a condition that rates little sympathy from those around you, but does provide them with continual opportunities for snarky remarks, and their full disclosure of old people jokes. This doesn't bother me because, as I'm usually the oldest in attendance, I'm smug with the knowledge that it too will happen to them. (Plus, as a lifelong smartass I'm due a bit of payback.) The real issue with hearing loss is that it tends to separate you from business and social circles. As it becomes increasingly difficult to understand what is being said, you tend to unconsciously avoid situations that point up your disability.

dilation in their blood vessels that, in turn, reduces the body's ability to cool itself. Regardless of the reasons behind it, it is not uncommon to hear an older rider say, "Man, I just can't handle the heat like I used to."

Skin, Your Largest Organ

It can consist of up to 10 percent of our body weight, is significantly heavier that our liver (our second-largest organ), can cover an area of more than 20 square feet, and is often the most neglected, abused part of our body. It is, of course, our skin. And yes, it is —by definition— a body organ as it consists of multiple cells working together to perform a specific function, or functions. Your skin's most obvious function is to keep your insides… inside. While doing that, it blocks pathogens (germs) from entering, helps to keep you warm by insulating, and cool by sweating, and provides necessary sensation feedback to the brain such as heat, cold, and pressure.

As riders, our biggest skin concern (apart from abrading it via asphalt) is skin cancer, the most common cancer here in the U.S. with

—according to the National Cancer Institute— more than one million people diagnosed each year. It is also the most curable of cancers if caught early enough. There are three primary types of skin cancer. The most common is *basal cell carcinoma* (BCC). While it is seldom deadly, BCC can destroy tissue and lead to disfigurement. The second most common skin cancer is *squamous cell carcinoma* (SCC), which can also disfigure. The most deadly of skin cancers is *malignant melanoma*, which causes an estimated 8,790 deaths per year in the U.S. It was not too long ago that the diagnosis of a melanoma cancer was considered a death sentence. Today, if caught early enough, this malignant cancer can be cured, but it does cause the majority of skin cancer deaths. Malignant melanoma cancer can appear anywhere in, and on, the body, whereas BCC and SCC are exclusively skin related.

While there are several behaviors that can lead to skin cancer, the most egregious one is overexposure to the UVA and UVB ultraviolet rays present in natural sunlight. And by the way, the artificial ultraviolet light used with tanning beds also poses a risk factor. While skin cancer is not specifically age-related, it does have a tendency to appear in older people, as it is a slow-growing cancer that usually results from years of skin abuse such as lengthy sun exposure, and sunburns. Since excessive sunlight is the culprit here, these three types of skin cancer types are more apt to erupt in areas that are continually exposed to the sun. Because of this, your face, neck, forearms, and the tips of your ears are particularly susceptible. Just how susceptible you are as a rider will largely depend upon how you dress. If all-the-gear-all-the-time (ATGATT) is your mantra, then you are minimizing your exposure to the UVA and UVB rays. If T-shirts and half-helmets are your style, then you are putting yourself at increased risk.

3 Additional Fun Conditions That Affect Riders of All Ages

Though not necessarily age-related, there are several other conditions that can adversely impact your riding fitness, and in some cases, quite possibly kill you.

Deep Vein Thrombosis (DVT)

According to the Center for Disease Control the average weight for a U.S. male aged 20 to 74 rose from 166.3 pounds in 1960 to 191 pounds in 2002. For females the numbers grew from 140.2 pounds in 1961 to 164.3 pounds in 2002. A November 2011 National Health Statistics Reports shows a further increase (between 2003 and 2006) of 3.7 pounds for men, and 0.07 pounds for women. I have raised the subject of weight because — in addition to contributing negatively to many of the ailments we've already discussed — it adds significantly to the likelihood of developing a deadly condition that is commonly found in adults over the age of 60: *Deep Vein Thrombosis* (DVT).

DVT results from the formation of a deep-seated venous blood clot (a thrombis) usually found in the legs. The primary danger with DVT is that the blood clot will break loose and travel to the lungs, brain, heart, or any number of other critical areas. When this happens it creates the possibility of a blood flow blockage that can damage organs to the point where death will occur. Generally, these clots are formed by extended seat time in a somewhat cramped position, which is why this condition is often called "Economy Class Syndrome" — and why it's of particular concern to us motorcycle riders. A high-profile example of death due to a suspected DVT was that of NBC reporter David Bloom, 39, in 2003. Reporting on the war in Iraq, Bloom had spent days in the cramped quarters of an Army vehicle. He had complained to military doctors about cramps in his legs and was advised to seek proper medical attention. According to reports, he took aspirin rather than obtaining the recommended attention and, as a result, ended up dying.

The only good to come from this tragedy was the heightened public awareness of DVT. David Bloom was an exception in that he was young, and not noticeably overweight, but his death serves to illustrate that a DVT can result at any age if the causative conditions are there.

With this in mind, consider the riding habits of many, both young and old. We often ride long hours in the saddle with the only minimal exercise coming every 100 to 200 miles when we stop for gas. Add marginal fitness and overweight to this and you can see where DVT could be a real possibility for many riders.

Carpal Tunnel Syndrome

Carpal Tunnel Syndrome (CTS) results from a pinched nerve in the wrist. More specifically, the median nerve that runs through the carpal tunnel at the base of the palm becomes compressed, usually resulting in pain, numbness and a burning sensation in portions of the hand. If left untreated, permanent nerve damage can occur resulting in reduced grip strength and continual pain.

CTS is an age-related condition insomuch as only approximately 10 percent of reported cases involve people under the age of 30. Generally, CTS is thought to be a repetitive motion condition, and is often thought of as a "computer disease" resulting from daily keyboard and mouse usage. However, there are several different factors that can cause CTS including, but not limited to, wrist anatomy (too narrow a carpal tunnel), prior wrist injury, and rheumatoid arthritis. There are also several non-computer related scenarios that can lead to CTS —such as repeated use of a jackhammer or other vibrating tool. Given that, it's not hard to see how long hours hanging onto a vibrating motorcycle can also be a causative factor.

In most riding positions, the carpal tunnel areas of both our hands are pressured by the grips. This can lead to burning, tingling, possible numbness, and quite often pain. This is particularly true of our left

and this... My DVT

My left arm had been bothering me for several months. Nothing major, just sort of a dull ache that was slowly increasing in duration and intensity. Having read all the warnings about how left arm pain can be a sign of heart problems, I reluctantly (remember, I'm a stubborn male) booked a visit with my doctor. An examination, and a resulting MRI showed that I had an 8-inch-long thrombosis forming in the brachial artery, which runs between the elbow and the shoulder. This was unusual in that DVT problems occur almost exclusively in the lower leg and thigh regions. As such, my condition had its own name, UEDVT (Upper Extremity Deep Vein Thrombosis). This is a nasty type of thrombosis because it has a track record that, in the words of the medicos, "has potential for considerable morbidity." In plain speak it means you can die from it. In telling me this I noted a bit of concern in my doctor's voice, which was justified when he stated that I needed to have that taken care of now. In most cases, DVT is treated with a blood thinner such as warfarin, or heparin, in a pill form.   ...continued

DVT *continued...*

My doctor felt that my case was severe enough to require surgery. The danger with UEDVT is that were a piece of the clot to break loose it can easily find its way to the lungs and cause a pulmonary embolism. This is a blockage of the lung's main artery, and not a good thing to have happen. The surgery took about three hours and was handled on an outpatient basis. It went without a hitch. I was placed on blood-thinning medication for several weeks and have had no problems since.

Given that I was not obese and quite active there was the lingering question of, "Why did this happen to me?" While the exact cause can't be determined, discussions with my doctor convinced us both that a prior break of my left collarbone (clavicle) had constricted the subclavian artery, which feeds the brachial artery wherein my UEDVT was formed.

hand, as it does not receive as much pressure-relieving movement as our throttle (right) hand. CTS is one of those injuries that tempts you to suck it up and tough it out. This is a capital-B Bad idea, as permanent nerve damage can occur which could lead to you being a motorcycle rider in your memory only.

Arthritis

Nothing screams Old Person! louder than arthritis. Arthritis is the inflammation and erosion of the connective tissue and cartilage surrounding our bone joints. While it can happen at any age, it usually appears in older people because we've spent a lifetime wearing away at our joints. If you've been active in physical sports, the odds are you've hastened the onset of arthritis by slamming into hard things (like the ground), and otherwise injuring your joints with tissue tears, overextensions, and fractures. According to the Center for Disease Control, in the period of 2010 through 2012, 52.5 million adults had arthritis in this country including 22.7 million physically limiting cases.

The two most prevalent forms of arthritis are *osteoarthritis*, and *rheumatoid arthritis*. The former is a degenerative bone disease characterized by the wearing away of the cartilage that caps each of our bones.

Rheumatoid arthritis is the inflammation of the *synovial membrane* that surrounds, lubricates and protects joints. Rheumatoid arthritis is an autoimmune disease that causes the body's normal immune system to turn against healthy tissue; in this case, the synovial membrane. Allowed to progress without medical attention, rheumatoid arthritis will lead to the erosion of the bone joints.

Arthritis can result from numerous conditions. Prime among these are normal wear and tear, broken bones, infection, and an autoimmune problem. It is possible, with proper medical care, to control the pain and stiffness associated with arthritis, but surgery is often inevitable if you want to maintain a high degree of strength and function.

Regardless of your physical condition, aches and pains can be considered a normal part of aging. As older riders, a long day in the saddle will usually remind us that our bodies have felt a bit of battering over the years. Hands can cramp, legs will stiffen up, and our backs complain. Usually, a few minutes of walking around, and a stretch or two will shake off these effects. If, however, you have persistent joint stiffness and soreness, you probably should talk with your doctor about the possibility of arthritis.

Now, The Good News! No...really!

That was a bit of a depressing laundry list of age-related problems, wasn't it? Not to rub it in too deep, here's a recap:
...and the bonus fun for *all* ages:

1. Brittle Bones (Osteoporosis)

2. Loss of Muscle Mass (Sarcopenia)

3. Balance Issues

4. Reduced Flexibility

5. Diminished Core Strength

6. Slower Thinking (Cognition)

7. Slower Reaction Time

8. Heat Intolerance

9. Impaired Eyesight

10. Loss of Hearing

Unless you are suffering from a debilitating illness, a traumatic

1. Deep Vein Thrombosis
2. Carpal Tunnel Syndrome
3. Arthritis

injury, or you've let the condition go past the point of no return every single one of these physical problems can be improved upon and, in some cases, reversed.

Of the 10 old-age ailments covered in the first part of this chapter, the first eight can be helped simply by committing to a regular program of exercise and proper diet. Let me drive this one home: no drugs, fad diets, or operations are needed. To limit your chances of acquiring an ailment that could keep you parked all you have to do is to get off your butt, start moving, and pay attention to what you are eating. The last two —eyesight and hearing— can be helped through early medical intervention. Even those three nasty all-age ailments listed under "bonus fun" can be improved upon with proper exercise and diet.

> *...every single one of these physical problems can be improved upon and, in some cases, reversed.*

Maybe You're Old Because You Want to Be

This brings up what might be an embarrassing question, but one you need to answer if you are serious about extending your riding career well into old age: Are you suffering from old age because you have to, or because you *want* to?

By the way, even that depressing bit of music quoted at the beginning of this chapter has a bright side to it. Here's the complete lyric:

> *"As soon as you're born, you start dying, so you might as well have a good time."*

5.

*In 2012, 43 percent of all motorcycle riders
who died in a single-vehicle accident were
considered to be legally drunk.*

Riding Stupid

If you ride while under the influence of alcohol or drugs — legal or illegal — you are... let me find the correct words here... being stupid. Or as my dictionary puts it, you are "lacking in common sense or intelligence."

During my years as the publisher/editor of *Thunder Press,* I received a significant number of death notifications that involved motorcyclists under the influence of alcohol or drugs. In 2012, according to the National Highway Traffic Safety Administration (NHTSA) 43 percent of all motorcycle riders who died in a single-vehicle accident had a blood alcohol concentration (BAC) level of 0.8 or higher and were considered legally drunk. On weekend nights, 64 percent of those who died were riding drunk. Polite society refers to these riders as riding "impaired." No, they weren't "impaired," they were stupid drunk, and they ended up stupid dead.

Despite the overwhelming evidence that drinking and riding can be a shortcut to assuming room temperature, many riders continue to indulge. We've all heard the reasoning, "I can hold my liquor," "I never get drunk," and of course, "I ride better with a few drinks in me." Stupid aside, riding under the influence of drugs or alcohol is a very selfish act because it ignores the painful and tragic consequences it inflicts upon others in the event of an accident; it is truly an "it's all about me" way of thinking.

If the statistics fail to impress you, or deter you from drinking and riding, consider how you might feel if you cause the death of another while "impaired."

My story:

It was August and I was on my way to Sturgis with a riding buddy, Rob. We'd added a couple of days up front for a quick tour of the Northwest, and on the third day we were in southern Washington. It was hot, and by lunch we were more than ready for a stop and a dive into a glass of something cold. Rob ordered a beer with his meal.

I'd made a pact with myself when I first began riding that alcohol, motorcycles and me would never find themselves in the same place at the same time. But with the beautiful scenery, great lunch, and hot weather, a beer seemed to be the ideal partner. I really wanted one. Fortunately reason took hold, and I reluctantly passed on the brew.

After a lengthy lunch we headed out. The area's two-lane roads meandered through beautiful country dotted with small lakes and even smaller towns. Just outside one of those towns I saw a man standing by the side of the road, just ahead of the car I was following. As I noticed him, he stepped onto the road from its dirt edge — there was no crosswalk. The car ahead slowed, but the man turned back to the edge, so the car sped up. I too had slowed down, but my gap to the car had narrowed. Just as the car passed him, the man turned and darted onto the road, directly in my path. I hit him.

The impact was hard and direct, hard enough to flip me upside down in the air.

The impact was hard and direct, hard enough to flip me upside down in the air. I recall looking back and seeing the man lying by the side of the road, up on one elbow, watching my flight. After that, most was a blur of frenetic activity mixed with pain.

My injuries were minor; ribs and a collarbone were broken, but nothing life threatening. The pain was intense though, so they doped me into unconsciousness for several hours. I awoke in a hospital room with a Washington State Trooper seated next to my bed. He seemed genuinely concerned about my injuries. With little preamble he told me that I held no blame for the accident as the elderly man had a habit of running across the road when traffic was present. He also told me the man had died.

The man had died. You cannot know how you'll react when someone tells you a person died because of your actions. I remember silence,
and my inability to say anything. The trooper took my hand, wished me
well, and left me stunned. I did not sleep that night.

Over the years I've replayed that day a thousand times in my head.
While I was "blameless," it was still my motorcycle that hit him. I have
dealt with this, and it is not my intent in telling the story to in any way
expiate my guilt. But I do have a point in telling. One of the thoughts that
crossed my mind in the months and years that followed was self-serving,
but contains a lesson: I did not have that beer at lunch. If I had, I would
forever be at fault not only in my own mind, but also in the mind of
others and probably the court of the authorities.

You indeed might be able to "hold your liquor," but if you injure or
kill someone after drinking —drunk or not— can you handle the consequences of your momentary stupidity? Can you handle being told, "The
man died."

6.

Motorcycling is not, of itself, inherently dangerous.
It is, however, extremely unforgiving of inattention,
ignorance, incompetence, or stupidity.

Anon.

Situational Awareness

Do an Internet search on "situational awareness" (SA) and you'll come up with a wealth of information, and more than a few different definitions. Many of them have a military origin, and most read as if they were written with the intent to obscure any message that the term might convey.

I came across one recently, however, that I find almost directly applicable to motorcycle riding. Interestingly, it came from a document related to the deployment of unmanned aerial vehicles (UAVs), or so-called "drones" which are commonly used in warfare and, now, by hobbyists and commerce. According to Major Brad Dostal, U.S. Army, situational awareness is: "The ability to maintain a constant, clear mental picture of relevant information and the tactical situation including friendly and threat situations as well as terrain." Translated from military-speak: having situational awareness means you know what's going on around you.

That sounds simple enough, and certainly obvious, but having full situational awareness while riding a motorcycle is a complex process that takes time and experience to master; it is a definable skill. For us older riders, it is also a skill that can diminish over time. When we were at the peak of our physical and mental condition, somewhere between 20 through 40, mastering a new skill such as riding was relatively easy. So easy, in fact, that we probably didn't realize what we were learning.

The truth of it is that actually, riding a motorcycle is the easiest part of becoming a rider, and that those physical activities — get on, start, go, and stop — are only a small part of becoming an experienced rider.

Let's go back and revisit Major Dostal's SA definition: "The ability to maintain a constant, clear mental picture of relevant information and the tactical situation including friendly and threat situations as well as terrain."

The key phrase in that definition is "clear mental picture." That is, a full understanding of what is going on around you. While the definition is applicable to our riding, it is incomplete because it does not reference influencing and/or controlling what is going on around us. We may indeed understand what's going on, but if we're only observing, rather than also participating, our best course of action would be to take the bus in place of riding.

What I offer here is a corollary: Situational Tactics (ST). This is the ability to understand *and influence* what is going on around us. So, where SA affords understanding, ST gives us the ability to participate in, and manage our riding. We really need both to competently operate a motorcycle.

Think of it this way, even if you understand what's going on with crystal clarity, if you only have situational awareness, but are not able to parse what actions you need to take in preparation for or in response to a situation, motorcycles aren't for you.

While riding a motorcycle there are three broad categories with which we need to be concerned:

1. Ourself
2. Our motorcycle
3. The road

In the following chapters, we're going to look at each of these areas with an eye towards their impact on us as older riders, and how SA and ST come into play.

"Situational Tactics (ST). This is the ability to understand and influence what is going on around us."

A doctor asks a patient:
  Sir, were you using a condom during the
    last time you had sex?
  Doctor, what do you mean by "the last time"?

Anon.

in other words

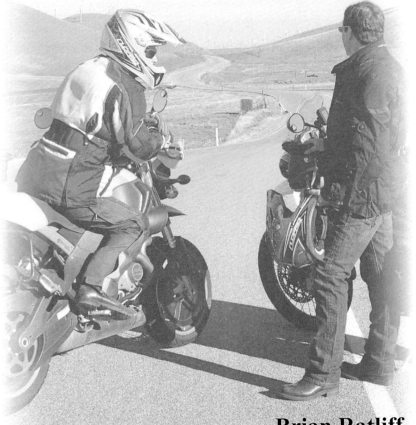

Brian Ratliff

Bob Gussenhoven

Brian Ratliff, 54

There are things I have learned I cannot do anymore

That license in my wallet, right next to my AARP card, says I will be 54 this year. I still remember lessons learned in a sand wash on a tired old Trail Honda. Thought I'd broken the sound barrier on an Italian Indian. Remembered almost not-soon-enough that early Bonnie's controls are backwards. Big old Huskys can pull wheelies in all gears. And if you can't start it you can't ride it.

There are things I have learned I cannot do anymore, and things that I should not do anymore. With age comes that knowledge; I will keep wisdom out of this. After a few too many mishaps at a younger age, no longer does the neck swivel like a teenager in a shopping mall nor do the ankles adjust to uneven

That license in my wallet, right next to my AARP card

surfaces like a parakeet on a perch. The back is a whole different subject, none really worth complaining about as one just learns to adapt and conquer. My body took the punishment of the years of toil and fun and now gives it back as a reminder to take it easier.

The most important thing is not what you have learned, but how to apply it. *Twist of the Wrist* by Keith Code is a great read. I didn't want to race but I wanted a better understanding of what I needed to know to safely push that line. Did I apply all of it to everyday situations? No, but it has kept me out of the radiator lane on a curve many a time by knowing I can push my bike a bit further and knowing it will not let me down, or put me down.

Many —too many— put their trust in a stranger to keep even minor things on their bike in check. I carry a tire pressure gauge and way too many times have told somebody that his or her front tire pressure looks a little low. And with an answer that "the dealership checked it just last week," I quickly offer to let them check it themselves; it awakens many to the fact that they should be a little more involved in the maintenances of their motorcycle. The only thing some dealerships really check is the proper deflation of your wallet.

I have found I do not need to be the first one there, though I usually am because I found the shortcuts years ago. I'm not afraid of a little dirt, even though my oil pan might not like it. Not all the great journeys can be had on a paved road.

Once in a while I get a chance to show up some fancy overpriced, overpowered beast of a machine in such a way that it get into the stories from days past. Never let a traffic signal catch you sleeping, and every intersection is a chance to work on your balance and slow racing skills. Keep up your skills or you lose them. When it is not in your heart to ride that day, listen to your heart.

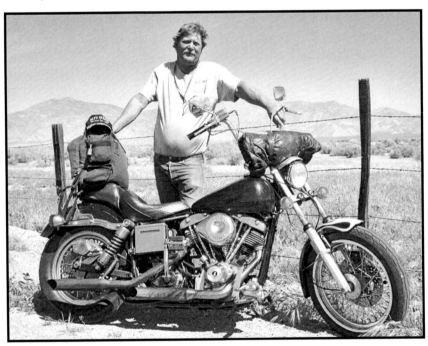

Bob Gussenhoven, 55

I began to feel like I was cheating myself

It seems to me that every rider evolves in riding style and accepted levels of risk. Both seem to run hand in hand as did mine. I started riding as a young man and have run the gambit of moto madness. By the time I hit my forties riding fast on the street was my style of choice, even while traveling long distances.

In my late forties I felt I was playing the odds like a gambler about to run out of luck. But I also began thinking, how long can I ride at this level of intensity before something major happens? The thought of waking in a hospital wondering what in the hell happened, not feeling my legs, and with the possibility of never riding again or —worse yet— dying and denying myself a full life of family and friends, is not I wanted in my future.

The decision to slow down came stubbornly. I thought maybe adding dual-sport motorcycles to my garage would slow me down. Not a chance; I reverted to my youth and rode like I was motocross racing. It took the cruel reality of a couple friends crashing and a major close call of my own to help me me see the light. I realized that I wasn't as sharp as I once was. Diminished judgment in all areas of control was evident.

Along with my newfound appreciation of riding and seeing the sights came a price.

This caused me to focus on destinations, and actually begin seeing some of the places I'd blazed through all these years. It's incredible the scenery you miss while traveling like you're on the last lap of a race. I began to feel like I was cheating myself out of all there is to see in the world. Finally, I gave myself permission to do what my mind and body have been telling me to do. Slow down a bit and enjoy the *whole* experience.

Along with my newfound appreciation of riding and seeing the sights came a price. A price I had not thought of: peer pressure. I hadn't considered this, and it was new to me. This caused me to make hard choices about whom I was riding with, and I found that riding by myself was actually fun. During group rides I started hanging back, enjoying the dynamics of others fighting for position. Having to explain why I no longer rode up front became easier as I better understood what I wanted out of riding, and the risks I was no longer willing to take.

Now that I'm part way through my fifties I have a better appreciation on what it is to be a motorcycle enthusiast. It seems that when you let go of the youth-filled narrow view of motorcycling, an entire limitless view appears. I'm certain that while the years continue to click by, I'll continue to be enlightened by what the sport and it's enthusiasts have to offer.

I currently ride a Triumph Tiger 1050 and a Suzuki DRZ400s. Neither is the best in its class, but both offer everything I need on two wheels.

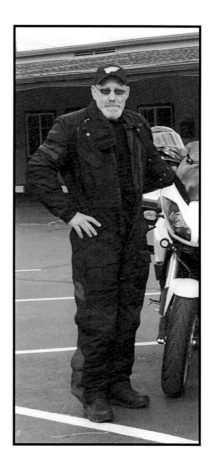

I have a personal trainer. She makes me chase rabbits
through the woods three times a day at a dead run.
Also, she has four legs and a tail.

Greg Tamblyn

TWO

do something about it

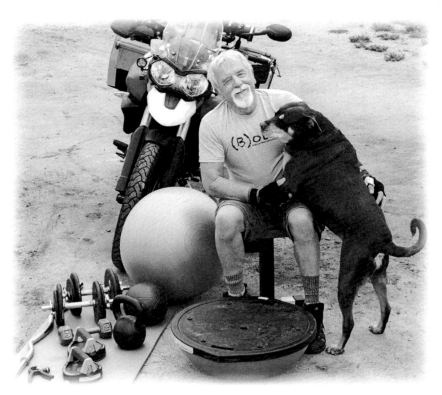

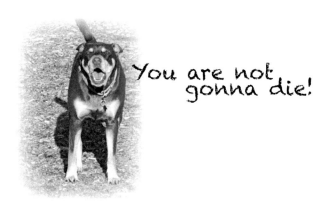

You are not gonna die!

OK… this is the obligatory disclaimer that can be found anywhere that suggests you actually *do* something.

Talk with fitness professionals and inevitably the subject of injury will arise, and generally they will tell you one of the primary causes of exercise injury is ego. And most of these types of injuries happen to …ready for the surprise? …men! Put another way, we men often believe we're more fit and stronger than we actually are. This error in judgment will often show up where weights are involved; using too much weight with too many repetitions. This results in strained —and possibly torn— muscles, back problems and a myriad of issues brought on by doing too much, too soon. Don't be stupid, check your ego at the door. Start your exercise program cautiously, and build it carefully.

Any physical activity can be dangerous to your health. If you are going to begin an exercise program, and/or follow any of my suggestions, the first step is to consult with your doctor. Tell him, or her, just what you have in mind. If you are in average health, a brief conversation might be all that's necessary. If you're overweight or have any breathing or heart issues, a test or two might be recommended. Typically, a stress test is given wherein you walk, or run, on a treadmill. This measures your heart's ability under a working load.

Take this advice and you'll rest easier knowing that while exercising you might feel like you're going to die, but you actually won't..

7.

I really don't think I need buns of steel.
I'd be happy with buns of cinnamon.
Ellen DeGeneres

What Does Fit Mean?

Everything in this book is focused on you (and I) becoming more "fit" riders. To accomplish this we need to begin with a definition: What does being a fit rider mean?

A very general definition implies being fit means we are able to live and enjoy our lives to their fullest extent. Now, let's narrow that down to the subject of this book; being a fit motorcycle rider implies that we can ride competently, comfortably, and for extended periods.

Riding Competently

The first — and most obvious — needed quality of a fit motorcycle rider is competence. We must have the necessary training, skills and experience to properly operate our motorcycle; that's a given. Also a given is that these competence skills are not constant and unwavering. They require constant attention and honing. There are many elements that can affect our motorcycle competence including our short-term and long-term physical and mental condition. For instance, if we tire easily our attention can wander away from the road, thus rendering us less competent — less aware — riders.

Riding Comfortably

Discomfort and pain are serious distractions. Lower back pain, for example, is a common problem with motorcycle riders. When we're suffering from tedious pain like that, our bodies can involuntarily tense up. This tenseness and distraction then negatively impacts our smoothness, riding precision, and enjoyment.

Riding for Extended Periods

One of the many pleasures that riding offers are the long trips to new and interesting places. If we're gritting our teeth half the time, fighting pain, trying to stay awake, and can't wait to dive into an Advil bottle, it's a pretty good indication we're not a fit rider.

Fit and Strong

While fit and strong are often used interchangeably, they have distinctly different meanings. We can be physically strong, but not fit, but we can't be fit unless we're strong.

Strong is the easiest to understand as it is usually measured in pounds; how many we can lift, pull, push, or carry. As this effort is generally of short duration, the aerobic factor usually doesn't come into play. That is, the condition of our cardiovascular system. Fitness —and general overall health— however, is ultimately measured by this system. If our heart, lungs, and the supporting network of arteries and veins isn't in the best of condition then neither are we, and how strong we might be is almost irrelevant in that we are not a physically fit person.

There is another important aspect to fit: It is specific. For example, a 300-pound NFL player can be very fit for a defensive lineman's position, but unfit to run back a punt. So, when I write "fit" I am specifically referring to our ability to competently ride a motorcycle during our old age.

Regardless of our needs, fitness results from three factors:
- Eating and drinking properly
- Exercising correctly
- Resting sufficiently

The amount of attention we pay to each of these factors is determined by what we want to accomplish. If our goal is to run a marathon we need to develop specific diet and exercise regimes that supports that goal. For our goal of being fit to ride a motorcycle well into our older years, our diet and exercise programs —while less stringent and strenuous than that of the would-be marathon runner— is still a critical part of achieving our goal.

If one or more of these fitness factors is missing, then we cannot become fit. We can lose weight, or we can become stronger, or we can be rested, but unless we have all three in play, we are not fit.

Function Follows Form

One of the unfortunate images that often come to mind when you think of an old person is that of a hunched over, shuffling along soul.

It's a pathetic image and too often a true one. Our spines are remarkable structures of vertebrae, muscles, ligaments, and nerves all working in conjunction to keep us upright and moving. Yet years of bad posture, bad diets and lack of exercise takes a toll on our bodies, bending us into an awkward shape that nature never intended.

In thinking about this I remembered a highway incident from several years ago. I live near the Salinas Valley, California's "salad bowl," a huge farming area supplying numerous fruits and vegetables to the rest of the country. Transporting this wealth of health from field to distributor requires a massive amount of wooden pallets. Ride anywhere around the Salinas Valley and you can't help but come upon flatbed trucks loaded with these, strapped securely —usually— in place.

I was on a back road that cuts through a large artichoke field. In front of me was a flatbed loaded with pallets. As I drew closer, it was obvious that the pallets were slowly shifting to the right. Not wanting to be a part of what I was sure was going to happen, I backed off. Apparently the truck driver saw what was wrong as he signaled to pull off the road. As his right-side wheels hit the rounded road shoulder the pallet load overcame the tie-downs, and tumbled off the truck. I passed without incident.

As his right-side wheels hit the rounded road shoulder the pallet load overcame the tie-downs, and tumbled off the truck

Think of your spine as that load of pallets, tied down by muscles and ligaments. As you move properly, your spine evenly distributes the load of your upper body across your vertebrae. Over the years, as our muscles lose their tone, and begin to atrophy, we have a tendency to hunch forward and our body shifts just like that load of pallets, and that nice upright posture that our parents taught us disappears, and in comes that awkward shape that nature never intended. The problem with this is not just that it makes us look older than we might be, but that it puts undue and unequal strain on our core and neck muscles.

To alleviate this strain, there are several things we can do. Foremost among them is proper exercise to keep our core muscles strong and flexible. When we're fit it's undeniably easier to keep ourselves walking strong with an upright posture. We also need to be aware of how we exercise. To keep our backs strong, proper form becomes particularly important when we exercise, and doubly so when it involves weights. As we get into specific exercises make sure to pay close attention to the notes on form.

The point here is that we need to actively watch our posture and form if we don't want to watch ourselves develop that shuffle that often requires one of those walkers with the tennis ball feet. We need to walk upright, walk proud, and slap ourselves when we start doin' that old-person shuffle.

Move It!

Our bodies are designed to move. We carry around more than 200 bones, 650 muscles, and 360 joints all working to keep us moving. Our arms are miracles of articulation, our legs incredibly strong and our backs supremely flexible. So what do too many of us do? We spend eight hours a day in a cubicle and too many hours on the couch… staring. And how does our marvelously designed body react to this? It shuts down. No, not all at once, but little by little. In fact we don't really notice it that much at first. We see it as an occasional sore, stiff back, and legs that don't feel quite as equipped to climb stairs as they once did. We write it off to age and take pride in the fact that we've earned the right to relax. My riding friends, this is called "whistling past the graveyard."

Our body is a complex system that continually monitors every physiological function. When this system senses a muscle that is not being used for extended periods, it causes the muscle to atrophy, to whither away. In effect it is saying, "Well, guess I don't need to bother with that muscle any longer." As discussed earlier this loss of muscle mass is called sarcopenia and, to a degree, is a normal part of aging; "normal" insomuch as this happens to a large percentage of our population, but not necessarily "normal" in the sense that we should think of it as an aging imperative.

We carry around more than 200 bones, 650 muscles, and 360 joints all working to keep us moving.

If you need a little more convincing, consider this: the January 2015 issue of the *American Journal of Clinical Nutrition* published the results of a 12-year European study involving more than 334,000 people. In its results, the study concluded that inactivity was killing twice as many people as obesity. They were not discounting the high morbidity rates of the obese, but concluded that (as quoted in BBC news) "The greatest risk [of an early death] was in those classed inactive, and that was consistent in normal weight, overweight and obese people." Note that this risk was present regardless of weight. And this from the study itself, "The greatest reductions in all-cause mortality risk were observed between the inactive and the moderately inactive groups across levels of general and abdominal adiposity, which suggests that efforts to encourage even small increases in activity in inactive individuals may be of public health benefit." In other words, just a moderate increase in activity can make a big difference.

I consider motorcycle riding a sport for five reasons: it requires exertion; not everyone can do it; it takes a learned, specialized skill set; it offers an endorphin high; and, done improperly, it puts the body at great risk. I'm not implying that everyone who swings a leg across a saddle needs to be an athletic stud, but to play our sport — that is to ride competently, safely, and for many years well into our old age — I am saying, not just implying, that our bodies need be in decent physical condition. And we can make this happen — not with a Spartan regime or the bench-pressing of small cars — but with the simple application of basic exercise, and a proper diet.

...the study concluded that inactivity was killing twice as many people as obesity.

Want to escape chronic pain and improve your riding? Stop blaming your unfit self on "normal" aging, take control of your day-to-day activities, and begin changing your aging self to your fit self.

USE It or Lose It!

The best exercise has nothing to do with health clubs, gyms, or slinging weights about. Instead, quite simply, you get the best exercise from living a healthy day-to-day lifestyle. There, I've just saved you buckets of money.

There was a time when the idea of a paying a business to allow you to exercise (and isn't that what a "health club" does?) would cause ample head scratching and probably a few laughs. But then that would be before we bought our food at mega-marts and our culture largely became the sedentary model that it is.

Somewhere around the mid 18th century, the Industrial Revolution kicked off wherein machines began to replace, or assist, people in the workplace. This usually made work easier, safer, and more productive. (High-fives all around for the Industrial Revolution!)

Though "industrial" has morphed into technology the revolution continues today as automation and computers push more and more of our population behind desks. The lifting, squatting, walking, and sweating that once comprised a big part of work has largely disappeared for many of us. This work-related exercise was once the norm and served to keep us fit. Today it is the exception. In fact it is such an exception that I've assigned it an acronym: USE, an informal shorthand for "UnStructured Exercise."

While USE sounds a bit contradictory it does serve to describe all the movements we make that aren't done in the name of formal, scheduled exercise. This includes things such as mowing the lawn, washing the car, walking the dog, and just moving in general. The critical aspect of USE is just that: It's critical. When you're dead you stop moving, but it is also true to say that when you stop moving you're on your way to dead somewhat quicker. As you move less your muscles disappear, your heart grows weaker and, eventually, your body's autoimmune system hangs out a sign that reads,

High-fives for the Industrial Revolution!

"Welcome to any and all harmful diseases and microorganisms and severe disability caused by simple injuries!"

To counteract the impact of the technology revolution — the internet, the television remote, the myriad selection of labor-saving devices at our beck and call, and our lack of USE — many of us join a health club, regularly pound the pavement with our running shoes, ride a mountain bike, and do whatever we can to add physical activity to our lives. All of this is good. As I've repeated many times throughout this book, physical activity is good and imperative if we want to stay upright, fit, and riding to the best of our ability for many years to come. The important take-away here is the idea that we need to keep everything in balance. A structured, scheduled exercise is excellent, but we need to also remember the importance of developing muscles in line with the way our body naturally uses them. In other words, mountain biking is a first-rate form of exercise, but don't overlook the importance of working the everyday muscles that come into play when we do USE activities like walking the dog, mowing the lawn and bending to wash the car.

Taking a spin class (stationary bicycle) so that you have an excuse to never walk anywhere ever again is kind of like stealing from Peter to pay Paul. You may become a great cyclist but your body isn't necessarily building up the muscles you need to do everyday tasks. Try to think of being active as a part of your life, and try to work in a balance of time at the gym (if that's your thing) and time for everyday USE activities.

There is no intent here to create candidates for the Senior Olympics. What I hope to accomplish is to point you in the right direction ... and maybe kick you in the butt a little... towards becoming a more fit motorcycle rider.

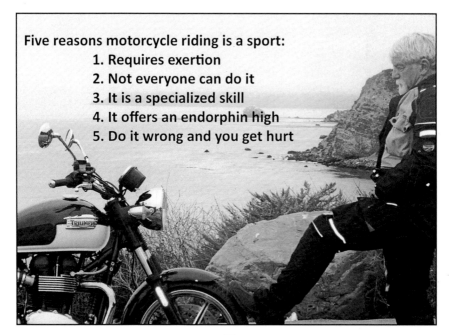

Five reasons motorcycle riding is a sport:
1. Requires exertion
2. Not everyone can do it
3. It is a specialized skill
4. It offers an endorphin high
5. Do it wrong and you get hurt

Being USE Full

Regardless of our fitness level we need to regularly review our USE activity. I've talked with several people who have cut back on their USE because they've joined a health club. This is a mistake because as beneficial as a health club can be, what with its myriad of machines and smiling helpful trainers, it cannot replicate, for example, the exercise received from pushing a manual lawn mower through tall grass, or painting a living room. Those activities —and the hundreds of others that constitute our lives— call into play dozens of different muscles that often get overlooked when following a structured exercise plan.

10,000 Steps

The linchpin of USE is walking, simply putting one foot in front of another as often as you can. Of all the types of exercise available walking is probably the most cost effective in that all you need is a good pair of walking shoes. And its benefits are numerous and well documented. Walking has been shown to improve cardiovascular health by lowering blood pressure, improve overall body tone and fitness, increase mobility, improve mood, improve memory and learning skills, and aid in getting a better night's sleep. You'll note that I mentioned nothing about weight loss. Walking and weight loss have long been synonymous, but clinical tests have shown that significant weight loss and walking do not necessarily correlate. Yes, you can lose some weight by walking, but if that is your goal, you'll probably be disappointed.

Research "walking" and you will always come across the 10,000 steps mantra. All cite this distance as a daily goal. It's certainly a worthy one, and a bit of a stretch

The linchpin of USE is walking, simply putting one foot in front of another as often as you can.

for most people, but there's no magic in that distance. In fact, the term originated in Japan in the 1960's as the name of a pedometer *manpo-kei,* which translates to "10,000 Steps Meter." The average stride length for a walking adult is 30-31 inches, which calculates 10,000 steps as being between 4.73 and 4.89 miles. This can be difficult to achieve on a daily basis, particularly if you work at a desk job. In that situation, you have to make a serious effort to rack up close to five miles a day. There are several strategies you can employ to help you build up the mileage.

- Commit to a before work and after work walk

    Doesn't have to be much, but you could easily
    add a half of a mile or more to your daily total.

- Park as far from your job as practical

    If you live only a couple of miles from your work,
    consider leaving the car at home. Anther good option
    is to use public transit.

- Use the stairs

    Elevators don't do a thing for your fitness.
    An added benefit with stairs is that when you walk
    down them, you exercise muscles not normally used.

- Walk at lunchtime

    Don't eat at your desk or the breakroom. Instead
    walk to a local park or other appropriate area. If
    you normally eat at a restaurant, take a longer route
    to it, or find one more distant.

- Walk during your breaks

    A short, brisk walk will do far more for your mental
    sharpness than a soft drink or coffee.

- Use a bathroom, copy machine, and water fountain

    that are farther from your desk.

For those who work in a less structured environment —work at home, retired, outside— the opportunities to walk, or walk more, are numerous. For me, one of my best walking incentives is my dog. Twice a day, morning and afternoon, she comes in my office and stares at me. If I don't respond she emits a low-level whine. This is the signal to go to the dog park, and results in adding at least a mile a day to my total and some needed exercise for her.

How to Walk

You've heard, "You have to learn to crawl before you can walk." Let me add this, "You have to learn to walk, before you can walk." You may think you know how to walk, but to achieve the most benefit from it there are a few things you should know.

First, walk with authority. If you are just beginning a fitness program, the mere act of strolling along is of benefit, but once you've passed that stage your walking should be brisk, with long strides, and your arms swinging freely at your sides. The idea is to give your muscles, your

heart, and your lungs a bit of a workout. It is not necessary to jog or run,
but after you're finished you should be
slightly winded, and feel the exertion
in your legs and your core muscles.

Secondly, watch your form.
Earlier I mentioned that we should
"walk upright, and walk proud."
When walking briskly that upright
posture should be modified a bit so
that you are leaning slightly forward.
Walking in this manner exercises the
core muscles, those of the stomach,
sides and back.

You also need to pay attention to the placement of your feet.
Ideally, each foot will point directly
forward as you walk. If your feet splay
outward (*overpronation*) or inward

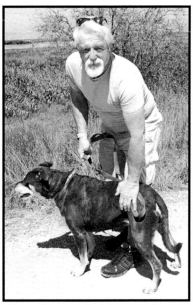

If you have a fat dog, you're
not getting enough exercise.

(*supination*) it can cause undue loading on various parts of your feet,
leading to ankle and foot pain. These two conditions are generally caused
by anatomical differences in the legs, the wrong shoes, and muscle weakness. This is one of those instances where a short talk with your doctor
could be of great help.

Thirdly, track your walking progress. Using one of the devices
mentioned in the "Tech Walking" sidebar, keep daily track of how much
you walk. While 10,000 steps is a worthy goal, that might not be practical for your current fitness level, or time available. The key to walking
your way to fitness is by gradually increasing your daily step count, regardless of whether your starting goal is 1,000 or 10,000. While that four
to five miles a day might seem like a lot, with a little determination on
your part —and employing some of the listed strategies— you'll surprise
yourself how quickly you can get to that level.

Swimming and Bicycling

I've put the emphasis on walking because it can be done by all of
us, most anywhere and with only a minimal outlay for a decent pair of
shoes. There are other forms of exercise that should be considered in

and this... Tech Man Walking

We are overrun with technology that seems to exist just because it can, not because anyone asked for it. Yeah, that's probably a bit of the old guy talking but having gone through the phase where I had to have every gadget made, I've found that, 1) the gadgets usually don't work as promised and, 2) even if they do, I really don't need them. Today I'm a lot slower at jumping on a tech bandwagon and because of this I've held off on using any of the very popular electronic "fitness trackers" that have popped up from numerous companies such as TomTom, Garmin, and FitBit.

At the same time, I do recognize that tracking my walking steps can be beneficial, as I need goals (and deadlines!) to motivate me. My first effort at tracking steps was a simple mechanical pedometer, and from that I moved to a hybrid electro-pedometer. I went through several of these, but I never really established the habit of using them. Two things got in the way. First, to gain the most benefit you should log your daily results; I usually forget. Secondly, I kept losing them! To work properly pedometers need to be clipped to your waistband or pocket, positioned where they unfortunately tend to inadvertently unclip too easily. Annoyed by the process, I gave up on this idea entirely until my wife Lora started using a FitBit.

There are numerous FitBit models. The model I use is called "One." It is small (2.25" x .75"), comes with a soft protective cover, and lives with me daily. Using it has become a habit because it overcomes the two issues I have with old-school pedometers: I keep the FitBit in the bottom of my pocket, which solves the loss problem, and the thing automatically logs its own data digitally, so I don't have to remember to do anything. Anytime I'm near my computer my step count is automatically updated. I also like that the FitBit shows distance, calories burned, and "Active Minutes." That last feature is important because those are the minutes of most exertion and, therefore, most benefit. There are several other features the FitBit tracks, including an all-but-useless sleep tracker (highly inaccurate), but step count is the most important one to me. ...continued

Tech Man Walking continued...

What I like most about this device is its unadvertised benefit: It nags at me. It doesn't beep or vibrate, or tattle on me to the world, but by

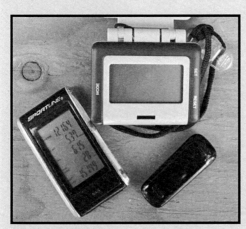

having a goal of 10,000 steps a day — and giving me my status on its small screen — it spurs me on to walk a bit further if I haven't yet made the goal for the day.

Just three of a multitude of fitness trackers. The FitBit is the small one at the lower right. The other two are some of the many I've tried, and discarded.

How it works

The heart of a FitBit is a 3-axis accelerometer. This is a very sensitive device that measures the frequency, intensity, and duration of movement fore and aft, side to side, and up and down. Then using "finely tuned" algorithms it converts this information to a digital readout.

So there, and aren't you glad you now know this. Maybe not, but here's what you should know: at times the FitBit is too sensitive. On a 300-mile trip with only normal gas stops my FitBit measured more than 8,000 steps. It is so sensitive —apparently— that it measures shifting, braking, and leaning motions. There are reports this also happens while driving a car.

addition to walking as they have their own unique benefits: Swimming and bicycling.

One of the many benefits of walking is that it has a very low physical impact on our bodies. If our ankles, hips, and knees are in good health walking does nothing but improve that health by building our muscles, keeping our joints loose and fluid, and properly exercising our tendons.

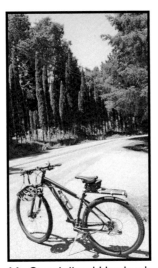

My Specialized Hardrock Sport with 29-inch hoops. Bad choice of wheels; smooth ride, but difficult to wheelie.

Walking is not, however, the lowest impact of exercises. That would be swimming. Additionally, swimming provides more of an all-body workout insomuch as our arms are usually exercised through the full 360 degrees of their capability. If you have ankle, knee, or hip problems, swimming is preferable as exercise as it takes the pounding away from these joints experienced while walking, minimal as it might be. I haven't put more emphasis on swimming because it is less available to most, but if a body of water is available to you, adding swimming can only benefit your overall fitness.

Riding a bicycle is also great exercise and obviously has a direct connection to riding a motorcycle as regards balance, the need to be fully aware of your surroundings, and the dynamics of two-wheelers. Bike riding is similar to swimming in that impact on our bodies is relatively low, which makes it a favored exercise with those suffering from joint issues. While it is excellent for cardiovascular health, it falls short in upper-body muscle building.

And then there's running

If you're a seasoned jogger or runner, you know the benefits that can be gained from this activity. It's great for overall fitness, in particular, cardiovascular health. So why haven't I put more emphasis on it?

I had a girlfriend in the late 70s who managed to coax a non-stop mile out of me; I've yet to forgive her.

Because, my old friend, running can raise hell with our body's joints.

When we're young, supple, and uninjured running can be a fun, beneficial way to exercise. We, however, are no longer young, supple is now a stretch goal rather than a given, and the odds are that somewhere along the way we either injured critical joints like ankles, knees and hips, and/or are suffering from underlying health issues such as arthritis or degenerative bone disease. Running is a high-impact activity that requires our lower-body joints to absorb and distribute the impact load every time a running foot hits the ground. Obviously, if the joints in question are not in good shape, this continual impact will work against fitness, rather than improve it. If, however, your doctor has given you the OK to trot forth I suggest you do it carefully as running can cause problems with our older bodies.

When I began this project of resurrecting my physical self I briefly thought of adding running to my exercise program. For most that might be a simple decision, but I've never been a runner or liked the idea of running. I had a girlfriend in the late 70s who managed to coax a non-stop mile out of me; I've yet to forgive her. In addition to having a strong aversion to running I've also suffered ankle injuries that make the idea, let alone the act, painful.

As my fitness improved I began to rethink this form of exercise, primarily because running is very effective at weight loss. Vowing to give it a try, I started with a treadmill but soon found that the ankle issue was a hindrance. Rather than give up the idea I began working on my ankle fitness. This mostly took the form of simple ankle lifts: up on the toes, back down. As time passed, I added a 20-pound dumbbell in each hand. Several weeks of this brought me to the point where I could use the treadmill without pain. From there I moved to the outdoors.

So, now I'm a runner? No. I call what I do "jalking." It is a combination of jogging and fast walking.

So, now I'm a runner? No. I call what I do "jalking." It is a combination of jogging and fast walking. Very slowly I'm increasing the jogging portion, but my pace is quite slow. I am happy, though, that I've broken down my anti-running stance.

Given the intensity of running versus walking it's obvious that running is superior in its ability to improve fitness, right? Well, not quite. There is ample evidence that the health benefits of walking are equal to, and in some areas, better than, those of running. In a 2013 study published by the National Center for Biotechnology Information, its author reached this conclusion, "Equivalent energy expenditures by moderate (walking) and vigorous (running) exercise produced similar risk reductions for hypertension, hypercholesterolemia, diabetes mellitus, and possibly CHD (Coronary Heart Disease)."

Running or Cycling?

What about running vs. cycling? In an August 2013 post on the *Men's Health* website they compared these two activities:

- Muscle-building

    They gave the edge to cycling with the proviso that you add in some upper-body strength work.

- Getting Fit Fast:

    Cycling won this one too. "Cycling's low impact, so you keep going longer," says Matt Parker, coach at British Cycling."

- Calorie Burn

    Running won this one. "Just 14.2 minutes on a treadmill burnt 200 calories. It took 27 minutes on a bike according to the Centre for Sports Science and Health study."

They had another interesting comparison. Under the heading "You want to stay off crutches," they noted that cycling had 6 injuries per 1,000 hours, but that runners suffered nearly twice as many (11) in the same amount of time.

So, do you walk, swim, cycle or run to get your exercise? My answer? Yes to all, in a perfect world. Just what you do should depend on your health, wallet, location, and the opinion of your doctor.

So, you think you're a runner...

The last day my brother-in-law, Jon Sutherland, *didn't* run was May 25, 1969. He was 18 at that time. He is now 64 and has run 16,797 days in a row. This has put him #1 on the list maintained by the United States Running Streak Association. (http://www.runeveryday.com/lists/USRSA-Active-List.html). Jon averages 11 miles a day and has run more than 192,000 miles.

Fortunately his sister, my wife, did not inherit that running gene. Had she, I'd be a great source of entertainment as she'd watch my attempts at running.

8.

I used to jog but the ice cubes kept falling out of my glass.
David Lee Roth

It's time...

The suggested exercises that follow require a minimum of equipment, are basic, and can be tailored to your degree of fitness. They are also very effective if you do them correctly and on a regular basis. They are largely anaerobic (strength training) as they target balance improvement and strength building by focusing on the major muscle groups: legs, hips, back, chest, abdomen, shoulders, and arms. However, as you increase the intensity and duration of your workouts significant cardiovascular (aerobic) benefit can be had. When you combine these exercises with an active USE regimen —particularly brisk walking— the result is a well-rounded exercise program that should help enable you to ride well into your older years.

How Much Exercise?

As to how much and how often we should exercise, the generally accepted answer to that comes from a government agency, The Office of Disease Prevention and Health Promotion. A report released in 2008 (Physical Activity Guidelines for Americans) recommends "for substantial health benefits" adults should do 150 minutes a week of moderate-intensity aerobic physical activity, or 75 minutes of vigorous-intensity aerobic activity. Additionally, the report recommends that this activity be spread out over the week (don't be that weekend warrior that ends up in traction on Monday). However, regardless of the level of activity it should continue for a minimum of ten minutes per episode. Examples of "moderate-intensity" exercise include brisk walking, mowing the lawn, and swimming laps. "Vigorous-intensity" activity would be things like running, mowing the lawn with a manual mower, bicycling at more than ten miles per hour, and jumping rope. Anaerobic exercise should be done a minimum of twice a week. While the report does not specify the amount of time you should spend doing this, the accepted wisdom is to exercise to the point where continuing would be difficult. In general, 30 to 40 minutes of anaerobic exercise is sufficient.

The big HOWEVER: The amount and frequency of exercise that you do is not controlled by a government report, but by your body. Previous injuries, your health, and your current state of physical fitness should all be considered when determining your exercise program. What is offered here are guidelines, and guidelines have never met you.

Exercise Basics

Exercise can be simple or complex, as determined by your physical goals. Just which level you choose will depend upon your starting point. If you've a desk job, prefer a horizontal position on the couch during the week and cram all your riding into a Sunday, your exercise program should begin at the simple end. That is, start paying serious attention to the USE part of your life.

If you drive around my small town in the early morning and late afternoon you'll notice any number of people attempting to push over trees, walls, cars, and similar large objects.

Warming up is an often misunderstood part of exercise. Essentially it prepares your body to exercise by increasing the flow of oxygen-rich blood to the muscles, which loosens and warms them up. This is important because cold muscles are more easily injured as they are less flexible and cannot absorb shock as easily.

Warming up should be done with a low-impact activity —and at a slower pace— for five to ten minutes. For example, walking, jogging (not running), or low-speed bicycle riding is excellent for warming up. If you are new at exercising it's recommended that you warm up for a longer period, as your muscles need to become accustomed to being used in a new way.

If you drive around my small town in the early morning and late afternoon you'll notice any number of people attempting to push over trees, walls, cars, and similar large objects. They are stretching before running off somewhere. For decades static stretching of the muscles was thought to be mandatory before any type of athletic activity. The theory was that in stretching the muscles it primed them for the activity to come. Claimed benefits of stretching included prevention of injury, and increased flexibility.

However, a highly regarded 2008 study out of the University of Nevada (among others) showed that stretching a cold muscle can actually have a negative impact on its performance that can last up to 30 minutes. Plus, stretching a cold muscle to extreme can tear it. Numerous other studies have shown no support for stretching as a way to reduce injuries. Lose the stretching part of your warm-up.

Once you've completed your exercise routine —we're getting to that— there is an equally important additional step: the cool down. During strenuous exercise blood rushes to the muscles that are under stress, and away from your heart. This is called venus pooling and can lead to dizziness and fainting. One of the primary reasons for a cool down activity is to assist the blood back into your full circulatory system. To counter the venus pooling issue a simple five-minute walk suffices. However, if you feel dizzy or faint, sit and rest till your body normalizes. Also, it is important that your body cool naturally; jumping in the shower is not the way to do it. In fact, doing that will often delay cooling as you will begin to sweat again after your shower.

It has long been thought that a cool down activity consisting of a gradual tapering off of whatever exercise was being down, resulted in the reduction of DOMS. Recent studies have shown that this is not the case as cool down has little or no impact on DOMS.

The only things missing from this kit are Moki (my dog) and my bicycle.

The exercises I demonstrate do not use all of these items as I wanted to keep things as basic (and inexpensive) as possible.

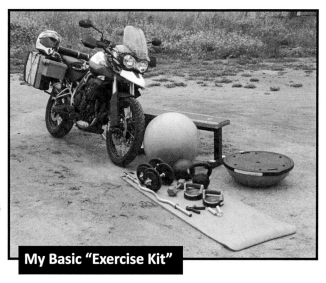

My Basic "Exercise Kit"

Stuff You Need to Know About Exercising

 Rep: A rep is a single exercise activity.
Ex: One push-up is a rep. Ten push-ups is 10 reps
Note: When the exercise includes separate action
by both the left and right sides of the body, 1 rep
includes both sides.

Set: A set is a complete set of reps
Ex: If you do 15 push-ups and stop, that is one set.
Two sets would be 30 push-ups with a rest in
between sets.

Routine: A Routine is a combination of sets.
Ex: Three sets of push-ups and three sets of
pull-ups would be a routine.

Hold: The amount of time you are to remain in position

 If you are new to structured exercise, or learning a new
one, begin with a minimum number of reps and a minimum
amount of weight. Rest between sets until you're
breathing easy.

 When exercising using weights, a *very* general rule of thumb
applies: To increase endurance, increase the number of
reps, to increase strength, increase the weight.

 Breathe deeply throughout all of the exercises. Do not hold
your breath. Breathe out when pushing or lifting, breathe in
when returning to start position.

Equipment You'll Need

Exercise equipment can be expensive; to fully equip a home gym
could easily set you back thousands of dollars. Then there's the
grassroots alternative that shows you how to make the needed
equipment at a fraction of the retail cost. (http://greatist.com/
fitness/21-diy-gym-equipment-projects-make-home).

I considered both the expensive and cheap options but, in the end,
I chose a reasonable middle ground as I —and you— don't really
need a complete home gym to achieve our fitness goals, and while
the DIY route was interesting, I felt it would detract from the purpose
of this book in that we're building bodies, not equipment.

The following is a list of the essential items I think you should have
to support your exercise program. Certainly there are options and

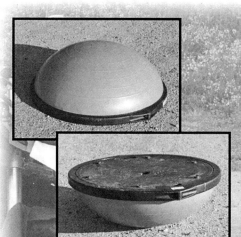

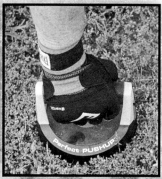

I prefer these stands for push-ups as they pivot on a base. This further relieves pressure on damaged wrists.

The inflatable "balance trainer" adds a balance and coordination factor to exercises.

If I were limited to four pieces of exercise equipment, it would be these. Used properly, they can work for an exercise beginner or the super-fit veteran.

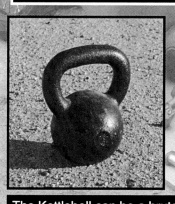

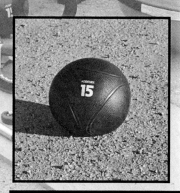

The Kettlebell can be a brutal piece of equipment. Start with a light one (10 pounds, for example), and use it carefully.

The Slam Ball is available in several different weights. As with the Kettlebell, start light.

alternatives to these, but this will give you a starting point. I have not shown prices because they can vary widely; shop carefully. Also, used exercise equipment is readily available with often —but not always— very cheap prices.

Walking / Running Shoes
> Why: The wrong shoes make essential walking very painful

Pedometer / Fitness Tracker
> Why: Great for goal-setting and measuring your progress

Bicycle & Helmet
> Why: Excellent, low-impact exercise

Exercise Mat
> Why: A sanitary, comfortable platform for floor exercises

Wrist Exercisers
> Why: Provides wrist-specific conditioning

Push-Up Stands
> Why: Relieves damaging pressure on wrists

Balance Trainer
> Why: A platform for strength and balance training

The items you purchase from the following list will be done by weight. It is important that you purchase weight that is appropriate to your physical condition: It is much easier to add weight than it is to repair torn muscles. All of these items are highly versatile when used with the equipment listed above.

Slam Ball / Medicine Ball
> Soft balls slightly smaller than a basketball. Available in numerous weights, generally between 4 pounds and 20 pounds. A good starting weight is 8 pounds.

Dumbbell Set
> Dozens of variations and weight combinations are available. I suggest a set with removable weights that total no more than 30 pounds each.

Kettlebells
> A stone ax-simple weight that is very versatile. Be careful about going too big here; you can hurt yourself, not to mention damaging walls, furniture, and bystanders.
> I suggest a 15-pound starting point. These things are ridiculously expensive, and shipping is not cheap.

The exercises that follow are, for the most part, very basic and have been tested by time. If you follow a regular regimen of strength training there are numerous health benefits to be had. According to the Centers for Disease Control and Prevention strength training "can be very powerful in reducing the signs and symptoms of numerous diseases and chronic conditions." Among them:

- arthritis   • obesity
- diabetes   • back pain
- osteoporosis   • depression

I've listed suggested routines at the end of this section.

The most difficult aspect of these —and all— exercises is sticking with it. Contrary to all the exercise happy talk that we read, getting— and staying— fit is not easy. Ya gotta work at it continually. Sorry, but that's the reality.

Let's start simple...

Wrist & Forearm   #1

Equipment:
  Wrist Exerciser
Reps: 10
Sets: 3

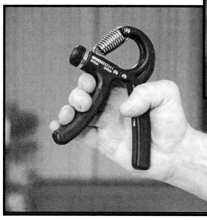

- Squeeze and release slowly
- Do not release completely; muscles benefit from continually being under tension.

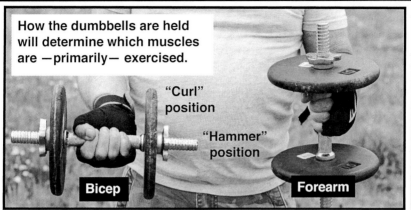

How the dumbbells are held will determine which muscles are —primarily— exercised.

"Curl" position

"Hammer" position

Bicep

Forearm

Equipment
Two Dumbbells: 10# each

Reps:
Dumbbells raised together: 10
or
Dumbbells raised alternately:
10 per side

Sets:
Biceps   2
Forearms 2

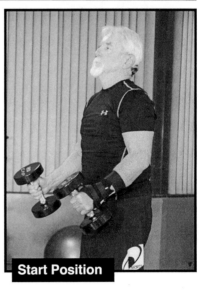

Start Position

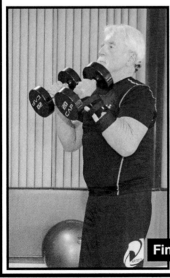

Finish Position

• Do not fully raise or lower weights;
keep muscles under tension
• Raise and lower weights slowly
• Back straight
• Knees slightly bent
• Feet spread to shoulder width
• Head up

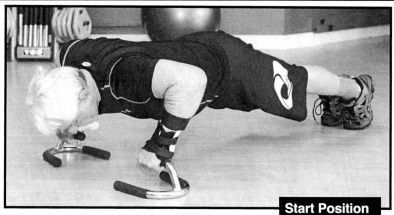

Start Position

Equipment
Push-Up Stands

Reps: 5
Sets: 3

• Raise and lower slowly
• Do not lower shoulders below elbow height
• Do not fully extend arms; keep slightly bent
• Keep back and legs straight

Finish Position

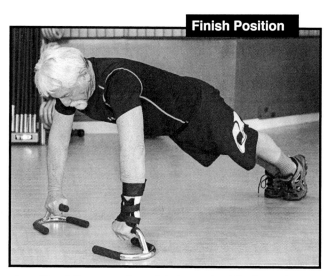

As with all the exercises it is important that you keep your stomach and butt muscles (abs and glutes) continually under tension as this helps to build core strength.

Equipment
Two Dumbbells: 10# each

Reps: 5
Sets: 3

Feet should be spread to shoulder width. Note that the dummy model did not do this in the "Start Position" photo.

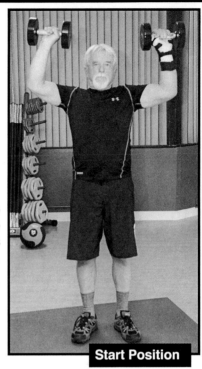

Start Position

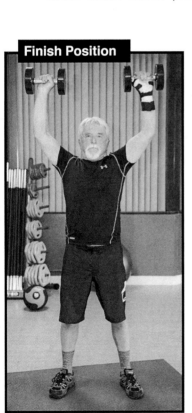

Finish Position

- Do not fully raise or lower weights; keep muscles under tension
- Raise and lower weights slowly
- Back straight
- Knees slightly bent
- Head up

Equipment
Kettlebell: 10#

Reps: 5
Sets: 3

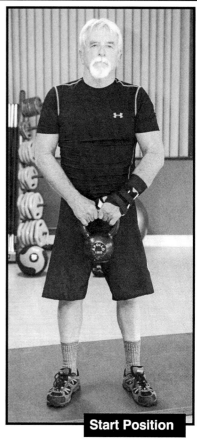

Start Position

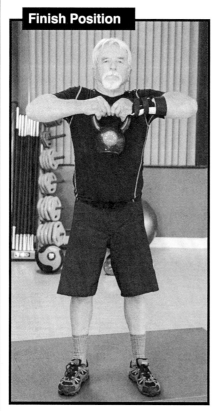

Finish Position

- Do not fully raise or lower weight; keep muscles under tension
- Raise and lower weight slowly
- Back straight
- Knees slightly bent
- Feet at shoulder width
- Head up
- Hold at finish position for 2 seconds before lowering.

Equipment
Kettlebell: 10#

Reps: 5
Sets: 3

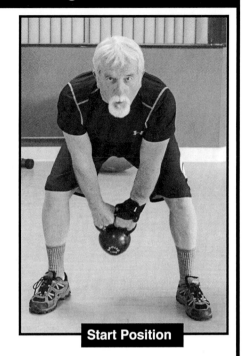

Start Position

Finish Position

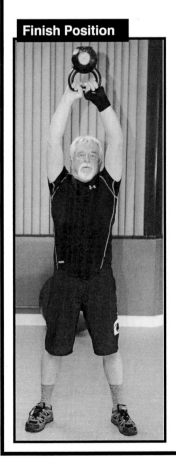

- Knees slightly bent
- Feet at slightly past shoulder width
- Head up
- Lower KettleBell between legs
- Gently swing KettleBell to overhead position
- Hold Kettlebell firmly; do not let it pivot in your hands
- Hold at finish position for 1 second before slowly lowering; do not let it swing down freely.

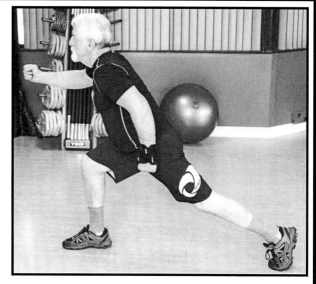

Equipment
(none)
   or
2 dumbbells,
   10# each

Reps: 5 steps
Sets: 3

From a standing position, take a long step, plant
your lead foot flat —hesitate— repeat.

As your conditioning improves, add a set of dumbbells.
Start with 10 pounds each.

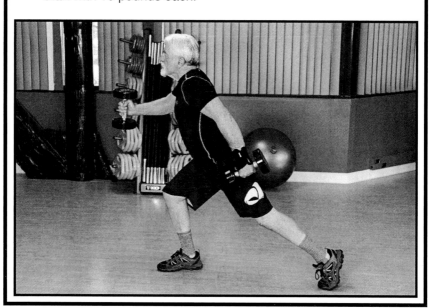

Equipment
(none)
or
2 dumbbells,
10# each

Reps: 3
Sets: 3

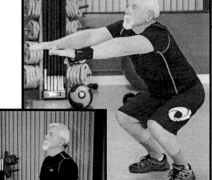

Start Position

• Do not lower butt past knee level
• Lower and raise slowly
• Back straight
• Head up

Finish Position

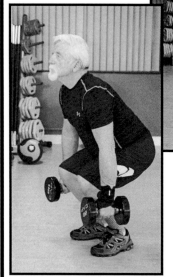

As your conditioning improves, add a set of dumbbells. Start with 10 pounds each.

Equipment

Matt
or
Matt and
Balance Trainer

Duration: 15 seconds
Sets: 3

This is a core exercise in that it impacts all the muscles in the central part of the body.

As your core strengthens, increase the duration. Get up around the two minute mark and you'll feel every muscle screaming at you.

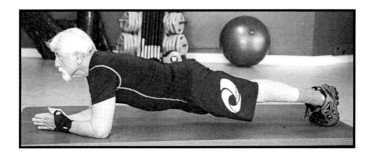

• Keep legs and back aligned
• Tighten stomach and butt
• Head up
• Hold position for duration

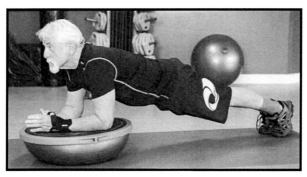

(hmm... unfortunate placement of that ball in the background.)

For variation, add in a Balance Trainer.
The movements of this half-ball further challenge your muscles and help to improve balance.

Equipment
(none)
or
Dumbbells 5#

Duration: 10 seconds
Sets: 3

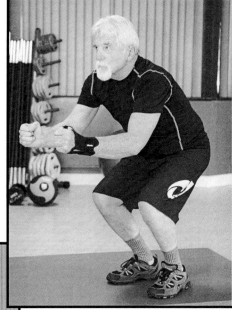

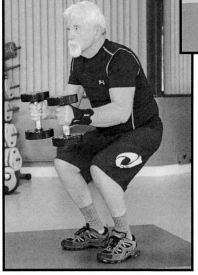

• Take a crouch position
• Hold for duration
• The lower your butt, the more difficult.
• Do not lower your butt below knee level.

• To increase difficulty, include dumbbells

For even more difficulty, stand on a Balance Trainer. The movements of this half-ball further challenge your muscles and help to improve balance.

Before trying this exercise practice with the Balance Trainer by balancing with both feet. Do not move on to the single leg stand (Stork) until you can balance easily with two feet on the Trainer.

Equipment
Balance Trainer
        or
Balance Trainer
Dumbbells 5#

Duration: 10
    seconds per leg
Sets: 3

Increase duration and/or weight to increase difficulty

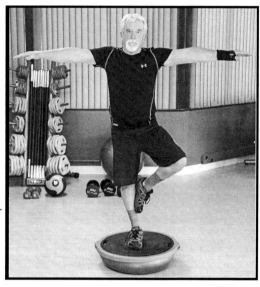

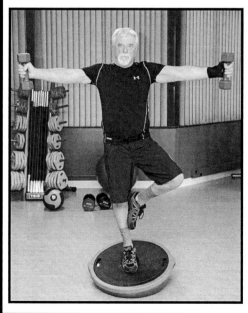

• Place foot in center of Trainer and slowly raise second foot and arms to positions shown
• Hold position for duration, dismount, switch leg positions, remount

Note: The weights in the lower picture are shown in the "Hammer" position. Rotating them to the "Curl" position exercises slightly different muscles. Get in the habit of alternating their position.

Before trying this exercise practice rocking the Balance Trainer side-to-side without using weights. Do not move on to the weights until you can safely rock the Trainer side-to-side.

Equipment
Balance Trainer
            or
Balance Trainer
Dumbbells 5#

Duration: 10 second
                      march
Sets: 3

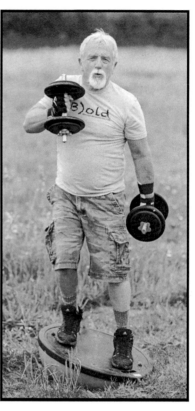

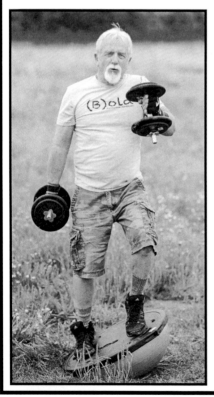

• Place feet approximately 3 inches in from each edge of the Trainer
• As you raise one arm push down with the opposite foot.
• Slowly march without stopping, rocking the Trainer side-to-side.
• Repeat for duration

I hate doing this exercise, but I really like how well it works on the majority of muscles, particularly the core muscles. While doing this you must maintain your balance, and focus on the moving ball.

As your body strengthens, you can change any —or all— of the variables: number of tosses, weight of the Slam Ball, height of the toss, depth of the squat.

Equipment
Balance Trainer
Slam Ball 5#

Duration: 5 Tosses
Sets: 3

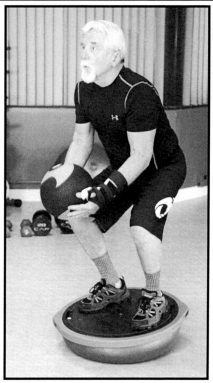

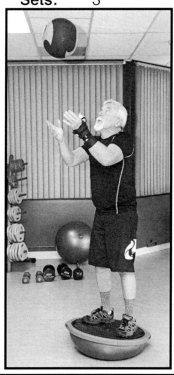

• Place feet approximately 3 inches in from each edge of the Trainer
• From a squat position, rise up and toss the Slam Ball in the air
• Catch the Slam Ball and return to the squat position
• Repeat, do not rest between tosses.

Do enough of these with a heavy ball and you'll understand why I named it "Upchuck"

...and what is that brace on my left wrist all about? Go to page 222 for the explanation.

Suggested Exercise Routines

The previous pages listed exercises #1 through #13

1. Wrist & Forearms
2. Biceps & Forearms
3. Triceps & Chest
4. Shoulders & Chest
5. Shoulders, Chest & Upper Back
6. Back, Shoulders, Arms
7. Legs
8. Legs
9. Core & Balance
10. Core & Balance
11. Core & Balance
12. Core & Balance
13. Core & Balance

Assuming three days a week of exercising, here are my suggested routines, by their number:

- Begin these exercises with the suggested weight and reps.
- Rest between sets long enough to breathe easily.

Day One: 2 (curl position) - 3 - 6 - 7 - 9

Day Two: 2 (hammer position) - 3 - 4 - 5 - 10

Day Three: 2 (curl position) - 3 - 5 - 8 - 9

- Once you believe you are doing these exercises with ease, add weight and/or reps, and decrease resting time between sets.

Exercises 11 - 12 - 13 can be phased into your routine only after you have mastered balancing on the Balance Trainer. Be careful, particularly when using weights, as falling off the Trainer is not unusual.

Exercise 1 should be done throughout the day. Carry the Wrist Exerciser with you.

and this... Aerobic vs. Anaerobic

Just moving is better than just sitting — without a doubt — but as you become more fit you will need to also become more selective in the way you tailor your exercise to better suit your overall fitness goals. An important aspect of this tailoring is understanding the differences between aerobic and anaerobic exercise.

Very simply, aerobic implies the "presence of air" and anaerobic the "absence of air." As it pertains to exercise, this means that aerobic exercise — usually referred to as cardio exercise — requires a heightened and prolonged use of oxygen to generate the necessary energy, while anaerobic activities can be described as any intense activity that is sustained for more than two minutes, regardless of whether or not you're out of breath.

All exercise starts as an anaerobic exercise, with only its duration and intensity changing it to an aerobic effort. Examples of aerobic exercise include endurance sports such as running, brisk walking, swimming, and motorcycle moto-X. Aerobic exercises are performed for several minutes, at least, and cause the heart and respiratory rate to elevate. Examples of anaerobic sports include weightlifting, sprint running, jumping, and any short duration, high-intensity activity. Anaerobic exercises are used to build strength and power, and draw energy from body chemicals rather than air. The good news is that both aerobic and anaerobic exercise burns fat.

"No Pain, No Gain"

"No pain, no gain" is often voiced by exercise buffs and athletes. It sounds very macho and all that, but taken too literally it can cause serious damage to any number of body parts. The idea behind it is that gains in strength and endurance depend upon working the body past its normal limits. For example, using our muscles within their limits can maintain tone and general fitness. To increase strength, however, muscles need to be stressed —worked beyond their normal limits— on a regular basis.

This stressing actually causes "microfractures" (also called, "micro-tears") in the cells of our muscles. Medically speaking this is referred to as *ultrastructural disruptions of myofilaments*. This is, to a point, a normal and necessary part of muscle building.

The downside of these microfractures can come as a surprise to those new at exercising strenuously—it's called DOMS. The "Delayed Onset of Muscle Soreness" hits the body sometime between 8 hours and 72 hours after strenuous exercise, and can feel like you've been beaten with a rubber hose. This soreness is a normal part of the muscle building and repair process and can reach painful levels.

However, it is critical to the health of your musculature to make sure that this soreness/pain does not turn into the pain that injures. As prevention of serious pain is a lot easier to deal with than repairing muscle damage, there are a couple of things to keep in mind. First off, if you experience sharp, serious pain —not just discomfort or stress— while exercising STOP whatever you are doing.

To push on through the pain is a mistake unless you are a trained athlete who understands exactly what the pain indicates.

To push on through the pain is a mistake unless you are a trained athlete who understands exactly what the pain indicates. Large muscle tears can take longer to repair than simple fractures; don't take the risk. Secondly, when working with weights a good rule of thumb is to keep the limit to where 10 to 12 repetitions tires the muscles to the point where rest is required, and increases to no more than 10 percent. For example, if you normally use a 50-pound weight in a given exercise, once your body gets used to that —that is, you don't experience DOMS— you can then in-crease that weight to 55 pounds. If you increase the weight by too much you risk damaging joints and tearing muscles (not the normal micro-tears). These types of injuries can take a long time to heal, and may cause permanent damage.

As an aside, I waited through a six-week recovery period for a torn lower-back muscle. The 10 days after the injury I was in pain enough to require a muscle relaxant and some serious drugs. This took the edge off but certain movements had me in a cold sweat yelling things best not mentioned in a family book. This tear resulted from my overdoing it with a back exercise, and ignoring the pain— lesson learned.

"I would much rather feel the physical soreness that comes with exercise than to feel the psychological soreness that comes with regret."

Steve Maraboli

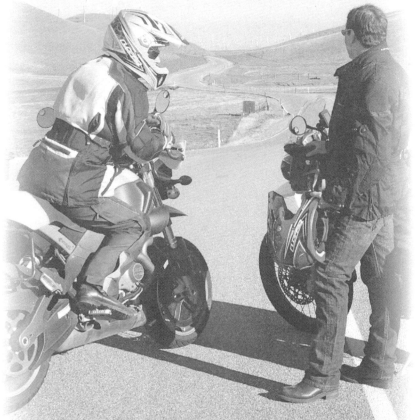

in other words

words

Bob & Sue Sgarlata
Susan Gore

Bob & Sue Sgarlata, 64 & 61

What We Know

What does it means to us to be riding our motorcycles over the age of 50 —or over 60 in our case? That intriguing question compels us to acknowledge that, regardless of our protest, riding changes with time.

The first change is instinctive and aptly memorialized in country singer Toby Keith's lyrics: "I ain't as good as I once was. But I'm as good once, as I ever was." Time wins all battles. The ticking sound gets louder; so we cherish every minute of saddle time. We begin to notice that we are not as quick, strong or as responsive as before, and on top of that we don't see as well. Sometimes, we kind of guess at what was on that sign we just passed. We gleefully ignore the laws of physics and the fact that we've lost some upper and lower body strength. We know that we need lighter bikes and shorter rides.

So what do we do?

We go out and buy more heavyweight baggers than any other age group, then add chrome, accessories, luggage and maybe a passenger and hit the road. We make longer road trips – and more of them. Riding off to more cool places, hundreds of gas stations, small town diners, national parks and monuments, hotels of every type, packing and unpacking the bikes. They don't make a bungee cord that can hold us. Sure we're over 50, but we have saddlebags full of experience and the know-how to make room for new friends, fun and memories. Let's ride!

We value every minute we ride because we know that the horizon holds more than the setting sun for us.

We finally know now what we didn't know then. We understand what it means to "ride smooth." We know when to let the speakers blast and when to listen to nothing but the sweet sound of a Harley. We know where and when to ride and where and when not to ride.

We know how to take a long trip with friends and still like each other afterwards. We know what to pack and how to pack it. We've learned to ride the right pace, to add bathroom breaks and avoid the interstate. We know to check for open gas stations before we hit the road in the middle of Montana, Wyoming or New Mexico.

We still believe that the journey is as important as the destination, but more than ever, we realize that arriving safely is more important than speed and ego.

We take time to take time. We sightsee and make photos stops. We treasure those pictures that we only have time to capture in our mind. Those are the ones that stay with us, and over time become more important than all those digital photos tucked away in our laptop.

We know a bike will be dropped and fellow bikers will rush to get it up and dust you off. We know that we'll never be able to control the weather or cars on the road; so we expect the unexpected.

We know more good roads than we will ever ride again; and that saddens us. We genuinely appreciate our beautiful country and how fortunate we've been to see it from the saddle of a Harley.

We still hope we know more than we did and less than we will.

We value every minute we ride because we know that the horizon holds more than the setting sun for us. When the time comes to forever leave the kickstand down, our only regret will be not riding more.

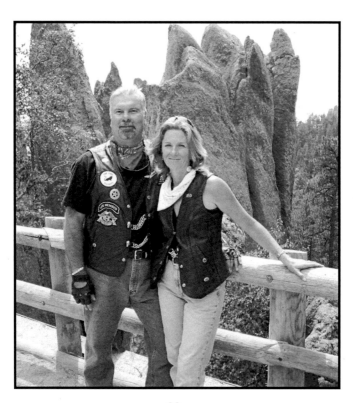

Susan Gore, 54

I have met some of the most interesting and endearing people through motorcycling.

Just a few months shy of my 50th birthday —and less than a year after my husband died— a good friend asked me to take a motorcycle training class with her. Recalling the time my uncle, a retired motorcycle sheriff, tried to teach me to ride a motorcycle (I was in my 20's) where I managed to run down a cyclone fence with him still on the back, and the few rides I had as a passenger while fixating on what my skin would look like in the event of a crash, I politely refused. I also reminded her that I did not have a motorcycle.

She informed me that the bikes would be provided; the course was a local fairground, that I would be doing her a favor, and it would be good for me to try something new. Ironically, she never made it to the course, but I did, and I took my 18-year-old daughter. What I didn't expect was how much I was going to love the way it felt to ride. Of all the people in our course, I had the least experience but the most fun, despite the fact that I was the only person to lay a bike down. I celebrated completion of the course by shopping for my first bike on craigslist.

As a woman alone starting into the world of motorcycles, the most helpful thing has been the strong support of friends who knew about motorcycles and riding. I needed to ride with other more experienced riders to feel comfortable. The kind of riders who have been riding and around bikes for more than 20 years and could tell

She informed me that the bikes would be provided; the course was a local fairground, that I would be doing her a favor, and it would be good for me to try something new.

the model of a bike at 150 yards going 70 mph. I found more good support within the motorcycling community. Harley and BMW dealerships will let you test ride their bikes (a near extinct customer service) and they have a strong network of group rides. There are also internet forums for riders; some with guided group events, beginner events, and women-only events. Being around riders with more experience gave me the information and advice I needed to feel confident enough to spread my wings.

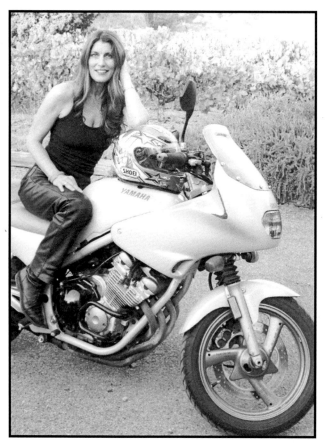

Best of all is to find a riding partner who lets you ride at your own pace and gives you room to grow without pushing. I have met some of the most interesting and endearing people through motorcycling. I wouldn't trade it for the world.

"Exercise is a great leveler. It doesn't matter how rich you are, you can't just buy your way into a great body. You have to do the work. I find that comforting. It's one of the few things in life where we're all on a level playing field."

Vinnie Tortorich

THREE

as we eat, so we ride

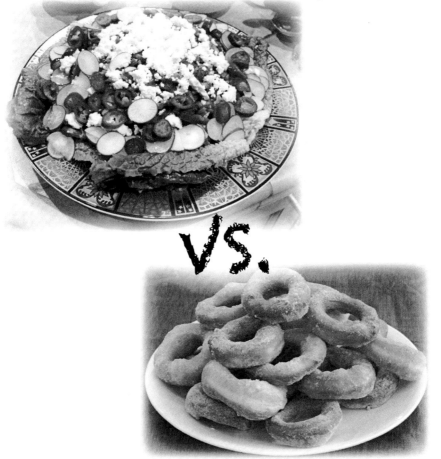

VS.

9.

A man walks into a restaurant and says,
"How do you prepare your chickens?"
The cook says, "Nothing special.
We just tell 'em they're gonna die."

Anon.

Food

From the start I knew that a section on food needed to be included in this book, even though I didn't want to go anywhere near the subject. Why? Because there are few things as controversial as diets, and it has become a complex, confusing subject.

Since their invention, diet books have been perennial best-sellers that merit their own dedicated section in bookstores. Why? Because there is a demand; we know we should eat properly, but we don't always know what "eating properly" entails. We're on a constant quest to find the diet program that will make us live longer, look better, and feel great. And, of course, most diets promise great results if we just follow *their* plan and not the dozens of other "great results" plans. So, we buy the book, sit down with a plate of nachos and a beer, and get about ten pages into it until it hits us: "uh…no."

Am I being just a bit facetious? Yep, but it's not because I don't take eating properly serious. You may have noticed that diet comes up in just about every lesson I have to offer about improving your ride. If we want to be truly fit riders we need to pay some attention to what goes into our mouths. Plain and simple.

In approaching this chapter I had to make a decision about just how deep I wanted to explore this subject. My goal here, as with everything in the book, is to give you useful information and to offer guidelines on how to apply that information to improve our riding fitness. It is *not* my goal to write a diet book.

What I'm including isn't revolutionary because we don't need a revolution to start being more aware of what we eat and how we eat. Take what I write as my opinion, but give it some serious thought. I am not a scientist, dietician or nutritionist, I am an old guy with a lot of years of experience who has been doing a pretty good job extending his riding career into his '70s. My hope is that this chapter helps you think about food in a new way.

How to Eat

Let's start with something that you may not have thought much about: how your environment affects what you eat.

Before I jump feet first into food and what we should eat, let's talk about some ways to approach eating. In particular, how to survive a few situations that beg for us to eat like it was our last meal. The interesting thing is, if you are prepared for these situations and you pay attention to just a few aspects that surround filling your face, you can significantly improve your diet without having to make any drastic lifestyle changes.

How to Approach Social Eating

Food is a great social lubricant. Arguments are settled over food, friends are made and, in general, life is a little better when you can sit down with enemies, friends, and neighbors over a good meal and maybe a bit of fermented beverage. This pattern remains a strong one today within our motorcycle community as "Live to Ride, Ride to Eat" is sometimes more than just a play on words. Group rides often start with a big breakfast, stop for a nap-inducing lunch, and then end with an epic dinner. The downside is that these group meals raise hell with digestion, diet, waistlines, and overall fitness.

When I'm on the road alone, my meals are simple and quick. If I'm camping — which I most often am — a typical breakfast is usually a single

...group meals raise hell with digestion, diet, waistlines, and overall fitness.

cup of coffee and oatmeal with fruit. Lunch will find me at a restaurant where milk, a small salad, and a pasta dish fill me. My dinners are back at camp and are usually of the dehydrated variety (chicken tetrazzini is one of my favorites). As my metabolism demands feeding every couple of hours, I consume plenty of apples, bananas, various trail mixes, and water between these three meals. Now, here's the telling thing about this diet: if my trip lasts five to six days, I will always lose at least two pounds, and yet have plenty of energy for long days in the saddle.

Contrast this with my eating schedule when I'm traveling with a group. For starters, regardless of the meal, they all take longer with a group. In fact, it's not unusual for just the ordering process for a table of six to take more time than it would for me alone to order and finish my meal. The problem with this is that extra time usually involves several trips to the antipasto plate and bread tray. Want proof of this? Ask yourself if you've ever filled up on appetizers before your meal arrived. Yep, me too. And then there's the, "Wow, that sounds good!" factor that comes with group meals. This is the moment where I've smugly decided on a baked piece of fish and a salad, and someone mentions french fries and a BLT and I start salivating. How about dessert? I seldom eat desserts, and actually have a fairly low craving for sweets. Invariably, though, someone will ask, "Anyone want to share some banana cream pie?" This is where my mind starts asking the question that never gets answered: Just how bad could half a dessert be?

One solution to this social eating problem is to eat alone. But a good life is more than just the food we eat. Some of my best memories involve overeating with friends. That's not something any of us wants to give up, so how do we balance a decent diet with the temptations of a fun group meal? Here are some strategies we can employ to keep our eating habits healthy and reasonable.

Social Eating Strategy #1: Talk About It

If you ride with a relatively small group (for example, six or seven people), you can bring the eating subject up ahead of the ride. Ask them to consider avoiding the fast food joints, and focus on restaurants with a wide variety of foods. You might be surprised to hear that your group agrees with you.

An even better option is to avoid restaurants entirely; purchase your meals from a market, and have an impromptu picnic. If you shop carefully (never shop hungry!) you'll be able to satisfy your hunger in a healthier, and usually less expensive, way.

If you ride with a large group such as a HOG chapter, getting all to agree where to eat can be almost impossible once you're on the road, so it's even more important to discuss this before the trip.

Social Eating Strategy #2: Keep to a Schedule

Most rides begin with food. For example, someone will suggest, "Let's meet for breakfast at 6 a.m." A better way to organize your ride is to say, "Let's leave at 7 a.m. Anyone who wants breakfast can get there earlier." This gives riders the option of arriving at the restaurant with enough time for breakfast if they want, but not enough time to fill the waiting time with unneeded pastries and sugared coffee. Another benefit of this is by stating a leave time, rather than an arrival time, you're more likely to get started in a timely fashion. And then, of course, there's this: Eat breakfast at home, then meet the group.

Social Eating Strategy #3: Pay Up Front

Unless the group has decided to evenly split the tab, one effective strategy that can help you watch what you eat is to request the bill as soon as you order, and to pay it when it arrives. Doing this can help you resist the dessert impulse. A side benefit is that it will help speed along the leaving process that so often gets bogged down when everyone tries to pay at once.

How to Avoid Overeating

Once your food sits waiting in front of you there are several additional strategies you can use to control eating more than you really need.

Consumption Strategy #1: Don't Leave Home Hungry

This is the simplest, most effective way to stop from overeating. Of the several fitness experts, dieticians, and nutritionists with whom I've spoken, most are in agreement that four to five small meals a day are preferable to the traditional three large meals. This is particularly true if you are very active. Our bodies need fuel to operate at peak efficiency and the amount of fuel we need is a result of calories expended, not the time of day. However (and isn't there always one of these?) if you have a well-regulated metabolism and function just fine on three square meals a day, there is no reason to change that pattern. Every person's need for food can be different — which, as it happens, is one main reason why there are so many different diet books, and why some plans works great for one individual and horrible for another.

On a typical day at home, I'll eat my first meal at about 6:30 a.m., my second one at 10:30, my third around 1 p.m., and I'll close the day off with a 6-ish evening meal. I carry various snack foods when traveling, with my favorites including bananas, apples, raisins and peanuts. As I generally stop about every two hours, munching on these reduces the likelihood that I will overstuff myself at the next sit-down meal.

Consumption Strategy #2: Be Conscious of your Meal Size

If you've traveled to Japan, you may have come across the term "American size." This refers to anything large and, in particular, the size of meals. In fact, we Americans consume the largest number of calories per person, per day, in the world: 3,770. In second through fifth place are: Austria (3,760); Italy (3,660); Israel (3,540); and Ireland (3,530). As a point of reference, most experts will tell you that active adults need no more than 2,400 to 2,800 calories a day to maintain their weight and energy levels. Because our bodies are quite efficient at dealing with food, the food that we eat beyond what we need to survive gets stored as fat. This is a genetic survival technique. Deep in our lizard brain we remain fearful that we'll starve if another woolly mammoth doesn't pass by again soon. To ensure our survival our brains tell our bodies we gotta store fat up to prepare for that coming famine. Fortunately, the food supply —(sorry, no woolly mammoths) in this country remains excellent, but, unfortunately, since our lizard brain doesn't understand that, it keeps storing away all those excess calories in preparation for the famine.

Possibly the best inadvertent diet advice ever offered came from the Roman comic dramatist Publius Terentius Afer (a.k.a. Terrence) more than 2,000 years ago when he said "modus omnibus in rebus." Roughly translated, (What, you don't speak old Latin?) that reads, "Moderation in all things." The next time you start to load your plate at the buffet table, think about your body storing all those dinner rolls up for the great famine and consider what old Terrence had to say.

Consumption Strategy #3: Illusionary Meals

In addition to self-control —which is sometimes hard to come by when confronted with delicious food— there are a couple of tricks you can use to control your meal size, particularly at home. You may not have heard of the "Delboeuf Illusion," but you've probably seen examples of it. This is where two identically sized dark circles appear to be different sizes because differently sized outer rings surround them.

What does this have to do with meal size? Researchers at Cornell University Food and Brand Lab discovered that people would under serve themselves when given a smaller dinner plate (Plate B) and over serve themselves when given a larger one (Plate A) because the larger plate makes the portion look smaller. Now hold that fact in mind, and add this one: Since the 1960s the size of our dinner plates have grown from an average diameter of nine inches to 11 inches in the year 2000. The bottom line: we are filling our much larger plates with more food than we need and it's affecting our waistline. When I came across this information, I immediately switched my plates: I now use our 11-inch dinner plates for salads, and our 8-inch salad plates for entrees.

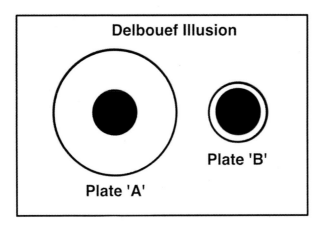

The dark circles are the same size on each plate, yet looks smaller on Plate A.

Consumption Strategy #4: Slow it Down

This is an eating trick you probably heard from your mother: Slow down! Don't eat so fast. There are several reasons to eat slower, but possibly the most important one has to do with two hormones, *cholecystokinin* and *leptin*. As we eat, our digestive tract releases these hormones into our bloodstream. Once these hormones reach a certain level our brains let us know, "Hey, you're full." The problem with this is that it takes about 20 minutes for our brains to process this hormonal information. In the meantime, we just keep eating. It's a bit like riding a train where the conductor mentions you should have gotten off two stops ago. By slowing down our eating we give our brain a chance to send that "full" message before we overeat.

Eating too fast and accidently overeating was once a regular problem for me. I'd wait so long between meals that I'd become ravenous, ready to eat anything I could get my hands on, and usually too much of it. When traveling, what I usually got my hands on was a cheeseburger, fries, and a large coke. I'd wolf these down, and then suffer for the next couple of hours.

Here's another bit of homespun advice that moms offer up: Chew your food 20 times before swallowing. I never really understood what that was all about — nor was it ever explained — but later in life I came to understand it. Obviously, the more you chew, the longer it takes to finish your meal, which helps you balance your consumption time with the 20-minute brain messaging time. Equally important, the more you chew, the longer the food is exposed to the digestive enzymes in your saliva, making digestion easier. Also, the smaller the food particles become, the easier it is for the nutrients to be absorbed before they pass through to your lower intestine.

Chew your food 20 times before swallowing. I never really understood what that was all about.

Consumption Strategy #5: Amend Your Family Dinner Routine

One of the enduring images of a bountiful life is the family gathered around a dinner table heaped with delicious foods. While this iconic imagery is indeed enduring, at times it can also feel illusionary as most families today find it difficult to gather the whole herd come dinnertime. There is an upside to this inability to gather your whole herd around for a traditional family meal, as studies have shown that a food-laden table actually makes it difficult for us to resist food that's right under our noses, and as a result, encourages overeating. The healthy solution to this is to serve food from the kitchen, then bring the plates to the table. (If you can get everyone in the same place at the same time, that is.)

How to Eat Right to Ride Right

Now that we've talked about how to eat, it's time to actually talk about *what* we eat. My guess is that this is no one's favorite part of the conversation. Stay with me. This part of the book isn't about pushing lots of carrots on you (although you should probably eat more carrots).

Rather, it is about helping you understand what food is and how much of what you need.

Have you ever asked yourself, "What is food?" Yes, it's stuff we eat, it keeps us alive, and pizza makes life worth living. But do you know what it is — just what goes into something that makes it "food"? Of course then you might ask, "Why should I care?"

You need to care because being a fit rider requires more than just physical strength and technical skills. What you put in your body has a direct effect on how well it functions. Bottom line? Eat right, ride right.

Food keeps us alive, but just how that works is where it gets interesting. To accomplish this staying alive thing, we need to eat at least a minimal amount of *macronutrients*: proteins, carbohydrates, and fats. Plus, we also require *micronutrient* minimums: vitamins, minerals, and water. And that, my riding friends, is the last opportunity for a group hug amongst nutritionists, dieticians, and diet book authors. Past this point the disagreements about what you should be putting in your mouth start to far outnumber the agreements.

As a basis for these disagreements, consider that a T-bone steak is high in protein, yet so is tofu. Bacon is also protein-rich, but then so is a handful of pumpkin seeds. Want a good dose of carbs? Most all candy bars will do the trick, but then so will dried fruit and wheat germ bread. And of course you must have fat to live. How about chocolate and fish oil? Or maybe pepperoni and Brazil nuts? Yep, fat in all of them. You can find diets that will include — and exclude — all of these items, and many other foods that can be given paralleled good versus evil arguments. Think about this, and you begin to see that the subject of diets can drive

What you put in your body has a direct effect on how well it functions. Bottom line? Eat right, ride right.

you mad. I'd like to save you from that madness, so what you'll find here is enough food information to a) get you interested in watching what you eat and, b) to set you on the right path towards a healthy diet, but not so much that this chapter will put you in the market for a straitjacket.

Fueling Your Body with Essential Nutrients

Food provides us with essential nutrients because our bodies cannot manufacture them or can only produce them in very small quantities. As noted above, these include:

- Protein
- Carbohydrates
- Fats

- Vitamins
- Minerals

Here's what each does, why you need them, and the best food sources to get them.

• Protein

What It Does

Protein can be considered our body's maintenance and construction nutrient, and is the primary structural component in all of our cells, in every body part, and in all of our tissue.

Common Sources of Protein

Milk products, meat, fish, eggs, whole grains, fresh fruits, nuts

And if We Don't Get Enough Protein?

Protein malnutrition can cause decreased immunity, loss of muscle mass, heart and respiratory problems, and even death.

• Carbohydrates (Carbs)

What They Do

Carbohydrates are the most important source of energy for our bodies. Our digestive system processes carbs into glucose (blood sugar), which is the fuel on which we operate. One of the key features of carbs is that this digestive process works quickly to create glucose and supply us with the energy boost we often need.

Common Sources of Carbohydrates

Carbs are commonly found in three forms:
Sugar. Sugar occurs naturally in many foods, including fruits, vegetables, milk, and milk products like yogurt and cheese. Unfortunately, we too often turn to what I call unnatural sources for our sugar intake like candy bars, soft drinks, and sugar-laden "energy" drinks. A good rule of thumb is to go toward the first category and limit your intake of the second.
Starch. Starch occurs naturally in vegetables, grains, beans, and peas. Starches are converted into glucose in our bloodstream. This is its sole purpose in our diet.
Fiber. Fiber occurs naturally in fruits, vegetables, whole grains, beans, and peas. Think of dietary fiber as a type of scouring powder for our intestines. Fiber is not digested by our gastric juices so it passes through our system absorbing water, and easing our bowel functions.

And if We Don't Get Enough Carbs?

Low blood sugar (hypoglycemia) is generally thought of as an ailment related to diabetes, but this problem can also happen in healthy people if the carbohydrate consumption falls below the required minimum. If you've gone too long without eating, you've probably experienced some hypoglycemic symptoms such as weakness, dizziness, headaches, or extreme hunger. That last one, extreme hunger, can cause us to binge eat, leading to weight gain.

Another potentially serious side effect of insufficient carbs is *ketoacidosis*. Without sufficient blood sugar, our body starts breaking down stored fat for energy, releasing ketone molecules into our bloodstream. To a point this is not a problem as it is a normal body function. It is only when the ketone levels become too high that we need be concerned as this condition can be fatal.

• Fats

What They Do

Dietary fats suffer from a bad name because, as we know, being fat is bad, so fat is bad, right? Well... yes and no. Carrying an unhealthy body mass is bad, this is true, but not all fats are bad. Our bodies actually require some fats as they provide energy and dissolve certain necessary vitamins. The problems arise when we don't recognize the difference between unhealthy fats and healthy fats.

Types of Fats and Common Sources

Briefly, there are five different dietary fats that we need to understand. The first two are the not-so-good ones:

Saturated fat raises total blood cholesterol level, and is also thought to be a contributor to cardiovascular disease and Type 2 diabetes. The primary sources of saturated fats are meat — red meat, in particular — and dairy products. Of course, you can also find data that refutes this. However, at this time the majority opinion supports reducing the intake of saturated fat. The U.S. Department of Agriculture recommends 12.6 ounces of red meat per week, My suggestion is to be aware of the amount of red meat you consume and if it exceeds that recommended amount consider chicken and fish as excellent alternatives.

and this... Sugar by any other name

According to the Harvard School of Public Health, the average American consumes 22 teaspoons (88 grams) of added sugar a day. In other words, sugar that is added to the foods we eat by the processors, and the sugar we add (to our coffee and cereal, for instance). This amounts to approximately 350 additional calories per day. The American Heart Association recommends no more than a daily intake of 100 calories of added sugar (6 teaspoons/24 grams) per day and warns that "there is no nutritional need or benefit that comes from eating added sugar." Added sugar is nothing more than empty calories.

It's easy to let your sugar intake get out of control, and even easier for sugar to put you on the wrong side of healthy. In addition to being bad for your teeth, putting you at a higher risk for cancer, causing addiction (yes, sugar is addictive), and directing you down the path towards obesity, sugar can also cause insulin resistance. Insulin is a critical hormone required for good health. It — among other things — allows blood sugar to enter our cells where it, rather than fat, is burned. Excessive amounts of blood sugar can cause insulin resistance that, in turn, stops our cells from accepting glucose. Having too much blood sugar (glucose) in our body can then lead to numerous health issues such as cardiovascular disease and Type 2 diabetes.

Just because it doesn't say "sugar" on the ingredients label, that doesn't mean that there's none in the food. In fact, added sugar comes in so many different names that you have to be particularly vigilant not to OD on the sweet stuff. Here's a list of different names for sugar that you should probably keep in mind when deciding just what to eat, and in particular, snack on. Yes, these are all sugar:

Barley malt syrup	Brown sugar	Carob syrup
Corn sweetener	Dextrose	Evaporated cane juice
Fruit juice concentrate	Fructose	Glucose
High-fructose corn syrup	Honey Invert sugar	Lactose
Maltose	Maltodextrin	Maple syrup
Molasses	Raw sugar	Turbinado sugar
Sorghum syrup	Sucrose	

Trans fat can be found in small amounts naturally in foods such as some meats, milk, cheese, and yogurt, but the primary source is man-made. Trans fat is created by adding hydrogen to vegetable oil (and referred to as partially hydrogenated vegetable oil), and is done to slow spoilage and ease cooking. The problem with trans fat is that it has been shown to increase unhealthy cholesterol (LDL) and lower healthy cholesterol (HDL), putting the consumer at risk for cardiovascular disease. LDL cholesterol has a vital physiological function in that it carries cholesterol to our cells for repair and maintenance purposes, but its level must be controlled.

And Now, the Not-So-Bad Fats

Monounsaturated fat (MUFA) is found in many foods and oils, particularly avocados, nuts, olives, and oils such as peanut and safflower. MUFAs are thought to improve our blood cholesterol levels.

Polyunsaturated fat (PUFA) is also found in many oils, in particular safflower oil. Also, decaffeinated espresso is very high in PUFAs. The danger with these fats is that they are unstable and can, for example, easily become rancid. Note that I've listed them under "...not-so-bad fats," and not "good fats."

Omega-3 fatty acids have both supporters and detractors, but the evidence on the good side is this type of fat can have beneficial results in a wide variety of areas, including cholesterol levels, joint health, mental health, and asthma. The downside: omega-3 detractors see less of the benefits, but don't find this fat to be harmful. The best source of omerga-3 fatty acids is fish.

What Happens if We Get Too Much or Not Enough Fat?

The biggest danger with too much fat in our diets is that it can dramatically increase the chances of developing cardiovascular disease and cancer. Interestingly, a study published in the March 2012 online edition of the *Journal of the American Medical Association* (JAMA) states. "Men and women with higher intake of red meat were less likely to be physically active and were more likely to be current smokers, to drink alcohol, and to have a higher body mass index."

• Vitamins

Vitamins are organic compounds required by our bodies. One use of vitamins is to regulate cell and tissue growth and determine how our bodies use minerals. There are 13 different vitamins needed by our bodies in order to stay on the healthy side of life, the majority of which are supplied by the foods we eat. Our bodies, however, naturally manufacture small amounts of vitamins D and K.

The vitamin supplement (pill) market is a $12 to $18 billion a year industry that has grown in excess of seven percent per year since 2009, and is expected to continue this growth into the foreseeable future. The two reasons for this are usually stated as, one, we are becoming increasingly health conscious and, two, the population of older adults continues to rise.

The majority of vitamins are sold over the counter, with no prescription needed and, in fact, are categorized as food not drugs. This is because the dosage size of these pills fall at or below what the Federal Drug Administration (FDA) says is the maximum dosage. This allows vitamin manufacturers to, at times, make exaggerated claims as regards to the benefits of their products. This, in turn, influences consumers, often making us believe that vitamin supplements are a necessity for a healthy life.

Do a bit of research, and talk with doctors and nutritionists, and you'll hear a recurring theme: A regular, balanced, healthy diet will provide all the necessary vitamins you need. No supplements are required. According to numerous credible sources, including the American Heart Association, the primary source of vitamins must be the food we eat, as it contains dietary components, such as fiber and bioactive compounds not found in pills. Additionally, vitamin supplements are often not fully absorbed by our bodies.

So why are vitamin supplements taken by at least half of our population? How's this for an expert opinion: "If vitamins were a regulated industry, megavitamins would have a black box warning on them," said public health specialist Dr. Paul Offit of the University of Pennsylvania. "We are the victims of an enormous marketing campaign."

Are doctor's that recommend vitamins quacks?

Let's back up a little bit. That some of our doctors might suggest vitamin supplements does not automatically place them in the quack category. The primary valid reason a doctor would recommend we take vitamin supplements is because we are not getting our requisite vitamins from balanced, healthy meals. This ties into the other reason for vitamin supplements being so popular: our ever-increasing population of older adults.

According to Donald McCormick, a PhD from Emory University, "A lot of money is wasted in providing unnecessary supplements to millions of people who don't need them." And he includes the elderly in his opinion. Yet, there are estimates that 50 percent of our population over the age of 65 takes supplements. Unnecessary? Largely. But, there are valid reasons for vitamin supplements. There are numerous medical conditions that

"Are doctor's that recommend vitamins quacks?"

can benefit from certain vitamins, and often the elderly have diminished appetites, leading to less healthy meals. Once again, let your personal physician make the decisions about your need for vitamin supplements.

• Minerals

Dietary minerals are necessary for health, and are classified as either macrominerals (needed in relatively large amounts) such as sodium, calcium, and potassium, and trace minerals (only small amounts needed) including iron, copper, and iodine.

Most everything I wrote about vitamins pertains to minerals also. That is, our primary source of minerals must be from the food we eat, and because the FDA considers mineral supplements food, they are not closely regulated. In fact, just about the only FDA requirement for both vitamin and mineral supplements is that they are safe; that we may benefit from them, or not, is not considered.

• Water

Keeping our bodies well-hydrated is often one of the most overlooked aspects of maintaining our health. We have a tendency to think of water as, well, just water. That is, nothing special, just something to quench thirst. Wrong thinking, dehydrated person!

Consider this: our bodies consist of mostly water, 50 percent to 70 percent in fact, and water is responsible for flushing toxins from our system, carrying nutrients to our cells, lubricating our joints, and regulating our body's temperature. To be healthy, we need to keep our bodies in fluid balance, wherein the amount of fluid we lose is offset by a like amount of fluid intake. So, just how much water do we need each day?

Looked at your pee lately? Well, you should.

On average, an adult living in a temperate climate going about a normal day's activities loses around 2.5 quarts (80 ounces) of water a day through urination, defecation, breathing and perspiring. Add in physical activity, and that water loss can increase significantly.

Keep in mind that these figures are not hard and fast for everyone, and that your fluid requirements may differ. But they do give you a starting point for determining how much water you should drink each day. Remember that old rule of thumb: eight glasses of water a day? Well, that turns out to be fairly accurate if you consider a glass to be eight ounces (8 glasses x 8 ounces = 64 ounces) and you add in the water intake from the food and drink you consume.

There is a quick test you can perform to see if your fluid intake is adequate: look at your urine. If you're peeing a close-to-clear, close-to-odorless stream, the odds are your water intake is adequate. The darker (and

"A key point about dehydration you wait until you're thirsty to drink, you've waited too long."

smellier) your urine, the more you are dehydrated, not to mention the possible presence of other problems. A key point about dehydration is that if you wait until you're thirsty to drink, you've waited too long. Dehydration can cause muscle cramping and dizziness; neither condition a desirable one while riding. This can be a particular problem for us older folks as we do not experience thirst as quickly as when we were young. The solution to this is to take regular drinks of water, even if you are not thirsty.

Hungry Doesn't Mean You Aren't Full

Once I began paying serious attention to what I was eating, I noticed how some foods filled me up quickly, while others left me still hungry. As I looked into the "Why?" of this, I came across the Satiety Index, as developed by Australian researcher Dr. Susanna Holt back in the 1990s, and published in the European Journal of Clinical Nutrition in 1995.

In her study, Dr. Holt fed 38 different foods to groups of volunteers. These foods were separated into six different categories: bakery products, breakfast cereals, foods rich in carbohydrates, fruits, foods rich in protein, and snack foods. Each serving of each food was 220 calories. During the test sessions, which lasted two hours, participants were asked every fifteen minutes how full they felt after eating certain kinds of foods. For the purposes of this study, white bread was used as a baseline. That is, in relation to eating white bread, how more or less full did a participant feel after eating other test foods. The data acquired from this study resulted in a Satiety Index (SI).

The highest SI score was that of boiled potatoes, and the lowest SI was that of croissants. In fact, the boiled potato SI was almost seven times greater than that of the pastry. Remember, each serving of each food was 220 calories. Translated, this means that the participants could eat seven times more servings of croissant (1,540 calories) to feel as full as one serving of boiled potatoes (220 calories).

A web-based nutrition center, Nutrition Data, took this and other information and developed what they believe is a more relevant indicator of fullness by incorporating the nutritional content of selected foods, which they call the Fullness Factor (FF). The higher the FF number, the more filling the item per calorie.

According to Nutrition Data, "Foods that contain large amounts of fat, sugar, and/or starch have low Fullness Factors, and are much easier to overeat. Foods that contain large amounts of water, dietary fiber, and/or protein have the highest Fullness Factors. These high-FF foods, which include most vegetables, fruits, and lean meats, do a better job of satisfying your hunger."

OK… so what does all this mean to us as riders?

It means that in order to feel full sooner (sated), we need to eat foods from the top half of the list (foods that contain large amounts of water, dietary fiber, and/or protein), and less of the items on the bottom half (foods that contain large amounts of fat, sugar, and/or starch). For example, we would have to eat three times more potato chips than carrots to feel equally full. This means, practically speaking, snacking during a gas stop should focus on, for example, apples and oranges, not candy bars. Note also that the top half contains more of what would be considered healthy, vitamin-rich foods, where as the bottom half is heavy with snack foods that are less nutritious.

Food	FF #
Bean sprouts	4.6
Watermelon	4.5
Grapefruit	4.0
Carrots	3.8
Oranges	3.5
Fish, broiled	3.4
Chicken breast, roasted	3.3
Apples	3.3
Sirloin steak, broiled	3.2
Oatmeal	3.0
Popcorn	2.9
Baked potato	2.5
Lowfat yogurt	2.5
Banana	2.5
Macaroni and cheese	2.5
Brown rice	2.3
Spaghetti	2.2
White rice	2.1
Pizza	2.1
Peanuts	2.0
Ice cream	1.8
White bread	1.8
Raisins	1.6
Snickers Bar	1.5
Honey	1.4
Sugar (sucrose)	1.3
Glucose	1.3
Potato chips	1.2
Butter	0.5

Making Healthy Choices

All right, you've read about how to eat, and now you have an idea what food actually is, so let's tie these together: What should we eat? Actually, the better question is, "How much of what should we eat?" To remain healthy, we need proteins, carbohydrates, fats, vitamins, minerals, and water, in the proper proportions as too much or too little of any one of them will cause physical problems.

Finding this proportion information can be tricky as there are all-to-numerous opinions and diets to choose from. I read through as

Guess who probably has the best nutritional information?

many of these as I could stand, but they served little purpose other than to confuse me. I did note, however, similarities in their recommendations. When I tallied up the common food type and portion recommendations that reappeared in every plan, I discovered that probably the best source for basic nutritional information was — surprise, surprise! — our own government.

In particular, the U.S. Department of Agriculture. The USDA suggests that our meals consist of foods drawn from five categories:

and this... Obesity

In July of 2014, U.S. News and World Report published this list of the world's most obese countries. A startling example of why "We're #1!" is not always a good thing.

1. United States
2. China
3. India
4. Russia
5. Brazil
6. Mexico
7. Egypt
8. Germany
9. Pakistan
10. Indonesia

"Obese" can be a controversial term, in that the condition is usually determined by a mathematical equation (weight divided by height squared) and not medical testing. All too often this gives people an open invitation to debate the validity of the math and create excuses about why the math doesn't apply to them. I can understand the controversy when the issue is normal versus overweight and it's only a pound or so that determines whether you fall in one category or the other. But when it comes to the "pound or so" that separates overweight and obese, the controversy should really quiet itself a bit since neither of these is a desirable condition. As it stands in 2015, obesity is currently the #1 cause of preventable death worldwide, and is directly connected to various diseases such as heart disease, Type 2 diabetes, and sleep apnea.

I'm not sure exactly where or when, but somewhere in our country's history we decided as a culture that "bigger is better" and I'm thinking it might be time to reevaluate that assumption. We've built — to name just a few — the tallest buildings, the longest bridges, and the biggest motorcycles. And today, we're building the biggest kids; in the past 30 years child obesity has more than doubled, and adolescent obesity has quadrupled. There are two reasons why all of the above is happening: 1) we are eating too much and, 2) we are exercising too little.

Vegetables
Fruits
Grains
Protein
Dairy

Here's the reasoning behind this, and (more or less) how much you should eat from each group.

- **Vegetables**

    Once again, our moms were right, and our Uncle Sam agrees with her. The U.S. Department of Agriculture recommends that half of our daily intake consist of vegetables and fruit. I'd like to define that a bit more. Of that half, put the emphasis on vegetables. Fruit is very important, but remember that the sugar content of fruit (fructose, the sweetest of all sugars) can be a problem if you overdo it.

- **Fruits**

    Yep, fruit should be our go-to snack and dessert, and a major part of our daily feedbag.

- **Grains**

    As much as possible, the grains we eat should be whole grains (as opposed to refined, bleached grains). That is, foods that contain the whole grain kernel, as these retain the most intact nutritional benefit.

- **Protein**

    Mention protein and most people will think meat — but nuts, eggs, beans, and peas are also excellent sources of protein. One important thing to remember when considering your meat intake is that the meats you consume should be as lean as possible. While that juicy cut of meat, ribboned in fat, may look delicious, it is not the healthiest way to eat protein; a better option is to trim the fat before you cook it or, if at a restaurant, trim it after your meal arrives and don't eat it. Another protein to consider is seafood. A good part of our meat intake should be at least eight ounces of seafood each week. Seafood is heavy in omega-3 fatty acid that can balance cholesterol levels and improve joint health.

- **Dairy**

    Milk and cheeses contain around 16 different nutrients, including significant quantities of calcium and vitamin D. The important thing with dairy products is to choose the low-fat variety.

If you would like to learn the nutritional makeup of the foods you eat, the USDA offers a 104-page PDF that will either fascinate you or put you to sleep. You can find it online at:

http://ars.usda.gov/Services/docs.htm?docid=6282

Food Summary

If you've read this far, congratulations! This is not the most exciting of subjects. Remember though, you've probably reached a point in life where paying attention to how and what you eat has a direct bearing on how you feel, and just how much more riding is left in your life.

As you've read, there is nothing particularly revealing or revolutionary about my eating and food recommendations. In fact, most everything I've written is really old news: a lot of which your mom probably told you. The idea here isn't to reinvent the wheel. Instead, the idea is to get you thinking, and part of that thinking process should be a serious questioning of what I've written. As I mentioned up front, diets are hugely controversial and some experts espousing their positions can challenge much of what I've written. That does not make the info here faulty, but it does serve to reinforce just how complicated the subject of diet can be.

Everyone is different, and while what you eat will largely differ based on your size, gender, activity levels, medical conditions and all sorts of other factors — two things will never change: a salad and an apple are better for you than a McDonalds hamburger and a piece of apple pie, and a meal that makes you energized is better than one that makes you feel like you can barely sit up, let alone ride a motorcycle comfortably.

Whatever diet you choose to pursue, remember...

Eat right, ride right.

Our bodies require 13 different vitamins to keep us healthy:

- **Vitamin A**

    Deficiency may cause night blindness and *keratomalacia*, an eye disorder that results in a dry cornea.

    Good sources of vitamin A include: liver, cod liver oil, carrots, broccoli, sweet potatoes, butter, kale, spinach, pumpkin, collard greens, some cheeses, eggs, apricots, cantaloupe, and milk.

- **Vitamin B1**

    Deficiency may cause *beriberi* and *Wernicke-Korsakoff Syndrome*. Beriberi affects the cardiovascular system, the peripheral nervous system, and other bodily systems, while Wernicke-Korsakoff Syndrome affects vision, coordination, muscle movements, and memory.

    Good sources of vitamin B1 include: yeast, pork, cereal grains, sunflower seeds, brown rice, whole grain rye, asparagus, kale, cauliflower, potatoes, oranges, liver, and eggs.

- **Vitamin B2**

    Deficiency may cause the mouth disease *ariboflavinosis*.

    Good sources of vitamin B2 include: asparagus, bananas, persimmons, okra, chard, cottage cheese, milk, yogurt, meat, eggs, fish, and green beans.

- **Vitamin B3** (also commonly called niacin)

    Deficiency may cause pellagra. *Pellegra* is a mental and physical disease with physical and emotional affects. The most common symptoms are diarrhea, dermatitis and dementia.

    Good sources of Vitamin B3 include: liver, heart, kidney, chicken, beef, tuna, salmon, milk, eggs, avocados, dates, tomatoes, leafy vegetables, broccoli, carrots, sweet potatoes, asparagus, nuts, whole grains, legumes, mushrooms, and brewer's yeast.

- **Vitamin B5**

    Deficiency may cause *paresthesia*, which is the scientific way to describe the tingling sensation you get when a body part "falls asleep."

Good sources of vitamin B5 include: meats, whole grains (milling may remove it), broccoli, avocados, royal jelly, and fish ovaries (oh yummy!).

- **Vitamin B6**

  Deficiency may cause anemia or *peripheral neuropathy*. Peripheral neuropathy is a nervous system condition that can cause weakness, numbness or pain in hands, feet and other parts of the body. Anemia is a blood condition that can make it difficult for your cells and organs to receive adequate oxygen.

  Good sources of vitamin B6 include: meat, bananas, whole grains, vegetables, and nuts. When milk is dried it loses about half of its B6. Freezing and canning can also reduce B6 content.

- **Vitamin B7**

  Deficiency may cause inflammation to the skin (dermatitis) or small intestine (enteritis).

  Good sources of vitamin B7 include: egg yolks, liver, some vegetables.

- **Vitamin B9**

  Deficiency may cause pregnancy complications linked to birth defects.

  Good sources of vitamin B9 include: leafy vegetables, legumes, liver, baker's yeast, some fortified grain products, and sunflower seeds. Several fruits have moderate amounts, as does beer. (You probably shouldn't consider beer an adequate nutritional supplement, though.)

- **Vitamin B12**

  Deficiency may cause *megaloblastic anemia*, a blood disorder that can cause anemia.

  Good sources of Vitamin B12 include: fish, shellfish, meat, poultry, eggs, milk, dairy products, some fortified cereals and soy products, and fortified nutritional yeast.

- **Vitamin C**

  Deficiency may cause *megaloblastic anemia*.

  Good sources of vitamin C include: fruit and vegetables. The Kakadu plum and the camu camu fruit have the highest vitamin C contents of all foods. Liver also contains vitamin C.

- **Vitamin D**

   Deficiency may cause the softening and weakening of bones, a condition known as *osteomalacia* when it affects adults.

   Good sources of vitamin D include: fatty fish, eggs, beef liver, and mushrooms. Vitamin D is also naturally produced in the skin after exposure to ultraviolet B light from the sun or artificial sources.

- **Vitamin E**

   Deficiency is uncommon. May cause mild *hemolytic anemia* in newborns.

   Good sources of vitamin E include: kiwi fruit, almonds, avocado, eggs, milk, nuts, leafy green vegetables, unheated vegetable oils, wheat germ, and whole grains.

- **Vitamin K**

   Deficiency may cause bleeding *diathesis* and *hypocoagulability*; ailments that can impact blood coagulation and cause hemorrhages.

   Good sources of vitamin K include: leafy green vegetables, avocado, kiwi fruit. Parsley contains a lot of vitamin K.

Courtesy of Medical News Today

http://www.medicalnewstoday.com/articles/195878.php

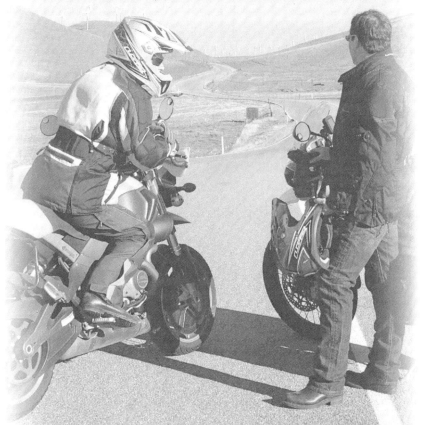

Ron Hilliard
Sandi & Will Long

Ron Hilliard, 55

Riding changes, but not the love of it

I got my first motorized 2-wheeled vehicle when I was 11 years old, a Bonanza mini bike. Coming from a family that was decidedly not motorcyclists, it was a hard sell to get my mom's approval, but I did succeed and it led to a lifetime of riding for me.

That little Bonanza gave me loads of freedom and made me feel invincible. I would crash that little bike and, other than some scrapes and bruises, be none the worse for the wear. I slowly graduated up through larger and faster bikes, always pushing the edge and inevitably crashing. Slowly those crashes began to hurt more and take longer to recover from. I began to realize that age was the culprit. Oh, and crashing.

Anymore it seems if I just fall over I get up with something broke and the prospect of long recovery times. Apparently old bones can be quite brittle. I'm also finding that the type of motorcycle that I choose to ride has evolved. Where I used to be drawn to the high-performance sportbike with all the capabilities of

I also believe that staying sharp and keeping those reflexes in top condition helps, but slowing down just a bit helps more.

killing me, I am now more drawn to the adventure-style bikes. I still like taking a super aggressive sportbike out for a little spin but now about a half hour is about all I can handle. Too stretched out and bunched up for my old muscles, tendons, and joints.

These days my primary bike is the R1200GS Adventure, kind of the big SUV of bikes. I find the ergonomics to be far friendlier to my aging carcass and I can still get plenty aggressive in the canyons, bringing back those feelings of youthful invincibility. I am also learning that I actually have to train my old body to get the full enjoyment of long-distance riding. It's not like I'm not fit, but I do find that my body just doesn't have the core strength needed for comfortable all-day riding.

I also believe that staying sharp and keeping those reflexes in top condition helps, but slowing down just a bit helps more. I no longer can react to the changes in conditions as quickly as I could when I was young and my eyes don't see is clearly as they once did.

I hope to be riding for a long time to come, but I also realize that as I continue to age the definition of riding will continue to change. I love the open road and I love being alone, but I have responsibilities to those who love me and plan on making sure that I don't do anything stupid that will bring my riding days to an end prematurely.

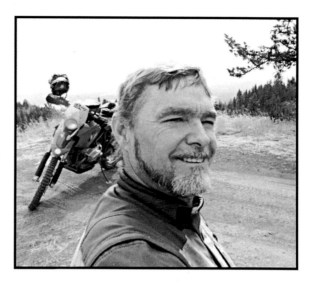

Sandi & Will Long, 72 & 71

They'll always find a way to ride

We started riding in our 20's in the 1960's. We've traveled thousands of miles together, cut the bucket list down one by one, and are still covering as many back roads as possible to get to our destinations.

How has it changed in our second 50 years as we age into our 70's (that just sounds old)? Not as much as you'd think. For us comfort of the bikes is more an issue now, where it wasn't in our youth; those bodies could take a beating. By comfort I mean things like handlebars that are set for us so that our old shoulders don't ache at the end of a long day, a clutch that doesn't cramp up arthritic hands. There are so many things you can do to make the bike fit you and be comfortable as you ride through the later years. By adapting our bikes and keeping our bodies as fit as possible, it works for us.

Do we stop more often? No we don't, in fact we might ride farther than we used to ride a Panhead and then a Shovel, and 100 miles was the limit. But with the bigger tanks, it's now about 125 to 150 miles between stops. But I do think we take longer stops, stretch our legs, hydrate ourselves much better and keep on our eating schedule as best we can.

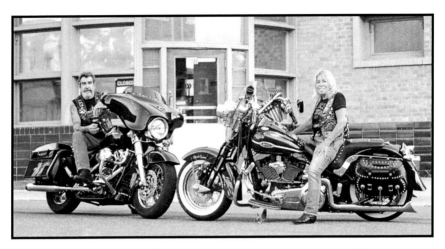

We exercise on a treadmill at home and on the road we try. We stopped sleeping on the ground at Sturgis in our 50's. We now get a room and get a good night's sleep. Rest is one of the best things you can do for your next day's ride. I must say, for us, as age creeps up, we haven't changed our riding all that much, but are trying to treat our bodies better, so that we can continue to ride into the sunset.

We know our years are limited and want to ride many more miles. Here in Idaho we don't have as many winter rides as we'd like, but if it's 40 and not too windy, and no snow on the road, we're out for a 50-mile putt. Our future probably holds a three-wheeler or two, when we can't hold up our heavy Harleys; it's still in the wind, so we're not against it. We might have to carry

We are a lucky couple, we love it together, and it has made life an adventure.

a few more pills, and complain about our aches and pains more, but it'll still be us, enjoying what we love.

Don't stop, find a way to make it work. We plan on many more back roads; our bucket list isn't done. Motorcycling is in our blood, no matter the age. It comes down to if you love something adjust to change, but don't give up. We are a lucky couple, we love it together, and it has made life an adventure. We have promised each other if one goes first, the other will continue to ride! Now get out there and get some wind in your face, there is nothing like it!

FOUR

the other part of fitness...

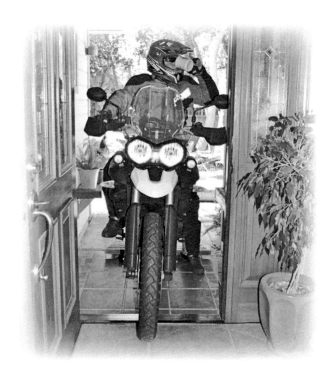

Being mentally and physically fit to ride a motor-cycle is the key to enjoying a long riding life. But maintaining that level of fitness is more than just eating properly and exercising regularly. We also need to put serious thought into the hardware and wetware end of things: our motorcycle, all those supporting items that make our rides enjoyable, and just where our head (that's the wetware) is at while we ride.

You'll find a lot of opinion and probably a basis for any number of good arguments in the following. As with everything in this book, feel free to fire back at me on our website:

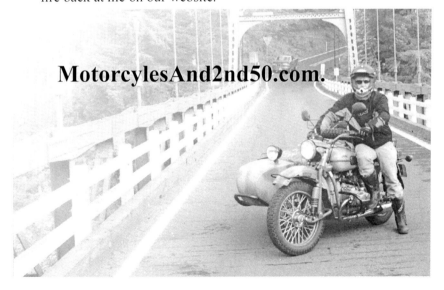

MotorcylesAnd2nd50.com.

10.

Q: *What's the difference between*
a Gold Wing and an Abrams tank?
A: *Oh about 40 pounds and a stuffed animal.*

Anon.

What We Ride

A s older, experienced riders we can remember when there were motorcycles... just motorcycles. If we wanted to tour, we strapped on a bedroll. If we wanted to race, we pulled off the lights. In fact, modifying our motorcycles for different uses was a big, expected, enjoyable part of the whole experience.

Today, there are touring bikes, sport-touring bikes, sportbikes, custom bikes, factory custom bikes, cruisers, adventure bikes, dual-sport bikes, naked bikes, streetfighters, street trackers, UJMs (Universal Japanese Motorcycles) and e-bikes — to name just the ones that come readily to mind. There are differences between these types of motorcycles, but at times those differences only add up in some marketing or styling equation, not functionality out on the highway.

Motorcycle marketing is intent on convincing us that a specialized activity requires a specialized motorcycle. I like as many motorcycles in my garage as possible, but I'm here to tell you that is a *want*, not a *need*. A cross-country trip *might* be more enjoyable on a Honda Gold Wing, or a Harley FL, but that shouldn't imply that not having one of those big

More important than what marketing thinks is what you think you should be riding. You need to put some serious thought into this decision.

guns means long trips are out of the question. A little research shows that almost every model of motorcycle ever imported has seen someone do extensive touring aboard it.

More important than what marketing thinks is what *you* think you should be riding. You need to put some serious thought into this decision. If you've been riding a while, you've probably graduated from one type of motorcycle to another. Possibly you started out on a sportbike, moved on to something a bit more comfortable such as a cruiser, and maybe you're now on a full touring rig. You've changed motorcycles because your needs and your idea of what's fun probably have changed.

As older riders who want to continue to ride, we need to carefully evaluate our motorcycle choices. Confidence behind the handlebars is essential for safe riding, and this confidence largely comes from being in physical control of the motorcycle.

Are you strong enough to ride your current motorcycle?

We need to be honest with ourselves: do we still have the physical strength to ride our motorcycle? And are we still enjoying what we ride? Dealing with the physical strength issue is relatively easy with a fair amount of hard work, as was shown in previous chapters. The enjoyment part? Well, that's a bit more involved. The question we need to answer is whether it is the specific motorcycle we're riding that's causing the problems, or whether we are burned out on riding in general.

Are You on the Right Motorcycle?

Starting with our motorcycle, we can begin to track down answers by asking a few questions. First, does the motorcycle we ride match our riding needs? It probably did when we first bought it, but how about today? Possibly that sportbike we purchased several years ago just doesn't fit in with our current-day touring plans. Or maybe that big dual sport is getting a bit tiresome on those long-haul freeway trips we're now taking. The most important thing is not to let our enjoyment be short-circuited by owning the wrong motorcycle.

Burned Out?

Tackling the other question — whether you are burned out on riding in general — is a bit more subjective. One complaint I've regularly heard is, "I have no one to ride with." As a rider who prefers solo rides my first thought is always, "So?" I don't voice that opinion because I realize for many the camaraderie of a group often outweighs the ride itself. If you're in that category, and for whatever reason your riding friends have disappeared, I can understand why giving up the ride might feel like a valid option. However, before you toss your helmet in the closet it would benefit you to search out new riding friends. One way to do this is as easy as a few keystrokes on your computer keyboard.

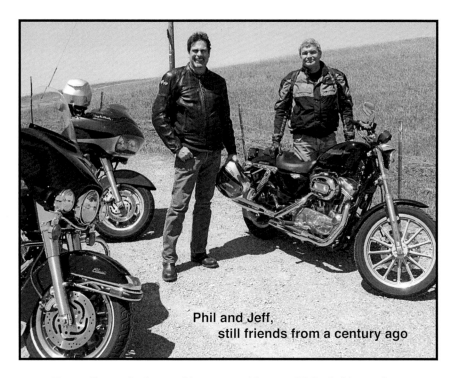

Phil and Jeff,
still friends from a century ago

Regardless of what and how you ride, you'll find riders of similar interests on the web. If you live in a heavily populated area, your choices of clubs, rides, and motorcycle events will be overwhelming.

For example, I typed "San Francisco Bay Area motorcycle events" into my search engine, and it returned more than 758,000 entries. Smaller town? OK, this time I entered "Baker City Oregon motorcycle events," and got back 112,000 entries. And yes, there are certainly duplicates among all those entries, but the point remains: there are lots of people to ride with out there! If you can't find anyone to ride with, well, you just haven't tried.

11.

Anybody can jump a motorcycle.
The trouble begins when you try to land it.

Evel Knievel

Gear Up!

Summer's uniform in the beach town where I live is a T-shirt, shorts, and flip-flops. Unfortunately, I often see that same style on motorcycle riders hereabouts.

The odds are that if you sport a minimalist style of riding gear you'll *probably* get away with it. That is, you might well have a long riding career without injury. But then again… you might not. Spend some thought on two words within that sentence; "odds," and "probably." No one can tell you the odds of not crashing, but I believe they are stacked against you. Accidents happen and the odds of you not having an incident at some time in your riding career aren't really in your favor. When this happens, your decision to ride in the muscle shirt and high-top sneakers will have painful consequences.

To the general public "road rash" sounds like something that might be treated with an anti-itch cream. We riders know that it's a bit more serious. In fact, it is often *very* serious. Road rash happens when your bare skins hits, then slides along, the ground and your top layer of skin — the *epidermis* — is ground away. To this point, it's the type of injury sustained on playgrounds and when one falls off a bicycle at low speed. The speed you were traveling on your motorcycle, however, keeps your body sliding which in turn tears all the way through your outer layer and into your

Road rash? More like road burn.
A reddish patch like sunburn = 1st degree burn
Tear off the outer skin = 2nd degree burn
Tear off the outer and inner skin = 3rd degree burn

inner layer of skin, called the *dermis*. And, of course, as you grind away at your body your open flesh picks up gravel, leaves, dirt, and anything else in its path. Road rash injuries are viewed and treated similarly to burns. If you've managed to come away with only a reddish patch similar to sunburn, it's called a first-degree abrasion (and you're very lucky). Tear away the epidermis and it ratchets up to a second-degree abrasion. Rip away the epidermis and the dermis, exposing fat, tendons, and muscles, and you've got a third-degree abrasion. Third-degree abrasions are very common with motorcycle accidents, and they usually require surgery and skin grafts that leave scars. All these degrees are painful, but second- and third-degree abrasions are particularly painful as they expose raw nerves. Now, doesn't that sound like fun?

And about those flip-flops. Talk to doctors and they'll tell you that foot and ankle injuries can be very difficult to fully repair. This is understandable as there are 52 different bones in each foot, and each connects to the fibula and tibia bones of the lower leg. And all of these little pieces are held together by a complex group of ligaments and muscles. The repair and healing of this critical mass of human wetware is painful, costly, difficult and lengthy. Serious foot injuries also tend to leave behind permanent damage that can result in a limp, a cane, or worse. Still want to protect your feet with a couple of layers of canvas?

Each of your feet contains 52 very vulnerable bones. And you want to protect them with a pair of flip-flops?

I could go on for dozens of pages outlining the gruesome results of inadequate riding wear, but I think you get the point. In fact, if you've been riding any length of time at all, you probably know someone that could serve as a very bad example of inadequate riding gear. Hopefully, you're not the example.

ATGATT

"All the gear all the time" (ATGATT) is a popular mantra among smart riders. It is difficult to argue with the logic behind ATGATT. That is, the more protection you wear while riding, the more likely you are to minimize serious injury in the event of an accident. Where the arguments arise is with the definition of "all the gear."

To many riders this means wearing a full-coverage helmet, a back protector, jacket and pants with full armor, over-the-cuff armored gloves, and tall boots made specifically for riding. There's little doubt that suiting up with this gear will better protect you in a minor to major get-off. You won't be invincible, but chances are good you also won't be holding down an ICU bed in the event of a crash. So, it's settled then; we're all going to be ATGATT'ed every time we get on a motorcycle, right? Right?

Well, probably not. Logic tells us we should wear all the gear, but reality often finds us less protected. We can probably agree that every item that is subtracted from the ATGATT list compromises our overall safety, so it really comes down to how much of a compromise we are really willing to make.

My riding apparel has evolved over the years from a simple leather jacket, open-face helmet, linemen's boots and leather work gloves, to most — if not all — of what's on that ATGATT list. This is particularly true on trips longer than just around town. On short hops I usually leave off the armored pants and back protector. Logically, that doesn't make a lot of sense, as I am probably more vulnerable in town traffic than I am out on the open road. Yet, spending ten minutes getting dressed for a five-minute trip to the hardware store doesn't sound right either. What often happens is that I, instead, say to hell with it and drive my truck.

Perversely, it seems adherence to ATGATT can reduce the amount of time you ride, but also significantly prolong the number of years that you ride.

The point here is that we have decisions to make before we get on a motorcycle. Each of us comes to those

---

My Basic ATGATT List:

- **Full-face helmet; Snell or ECE rated**
- **Armored jacket and pants**
- **Armored gloves**
- **Tall, buckle riding boots**

Optional:
- **Back protector**

Riding with anything less than these items compromises my safety. Do I do that?
Yes, I'll occasionally ride without armored pants, and sometimes use a lightweight pair of gloves, but I never forget I'm dancing with the devil.

---

decisions from different angles. My dirt track and roadracing experience strongly influences what I wear. Yet we all know many riders whose "uniform" consists of nothing more than basic street clothes and a barely legal helmet. However, as older motorcycle riders, we don't bounce — or bounce back — like we did in our 20's, and our bodies are not as resilient as they once were.

It's your hide, so it's your choice. But if staying on the road in one piece well into your 70's is a priority, you may want to reconsider your idea of "all the gear," especially if you're a T-shirt and high-tops rider. Your epidermis will thank you!

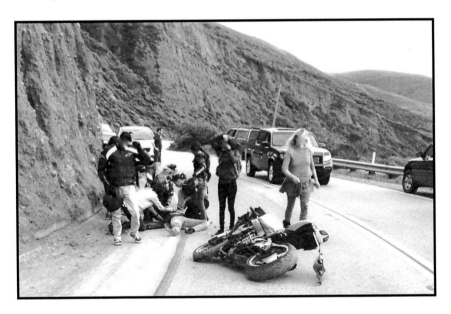

Yes, it happens. This was on the famed and unforgiving Highway 1, south of Monterey, California. Jeans and tennis shoes made it all the worse. This rider was one of a group of ten that passed me, across a double yellow line, at a very high rate of speed. I came on this scene about five minutes after that pass.

Helmets

Motorcycle helmets are relatively simple devices, consisting of —primarily— an external shell, an internal impact-absorption layer, a comfort liner, and a chinstrap. Every legal helmet sold in this country is built with those same components and every legal helmet sold in this country must meet the exact same test standards.

What this strongly implies is that regardless of price and regardless of manufacturer, no one legal helmet —of the same style— is more or less safe than any of the others. Am I saying that a $100 Snell-approved helmet is as safe as a $700 Snell-approved helmet? Yes, I am. I say this because I've not seen any evidence to the contrary. Marketing obscures this fact by often showing professional racers using their products. The idea is that if the helmet is good enough for someone risking his or her neck on a racetrack, then it's good enough for the general public. That a relatively few helmet companies use professional riders does not mean their helmets are safer; it means they can afford to sponsor racers.

Am I saying that there are no substantive differences with helmets? No, but it's worth mentioning that the differences that exist are not related to how protective a helmet might be. Instead the differences in price can largely be accounted for by graphics, the materials used in the comfort liner, and the face shield and venting assemblies. Manufacturing quality can also be a factor, though I have seen lower-end helmets with excellent

"...no one legal helmet —of the same style— is more or less safe than any of the others."

quality. Shell material can also impact price. In general, helmets at the lower end of the price spectrum have shells molded from various thermo-plastics, while upper end helmets are fitted with fiberglass shells. Again, there is no evidence to support that either material is superior as regards protection from impact. Remember, they both must meet the same legal standards.

At the very top end of helmet pricing you will find the shells made from some of the more exotic materials such as carbon fiber and Kevlar. Once again… safer? Highly doubtful, but they do have the advantage of lighter weight, and the disadvantage of premium pricing.

How a Helmet Works

A motorcycle helmet works properly if it is destroyed. Most riders believe it is a helmet's job to resist impact. Nope. A helmet's Job #1 is to absorb and disperse impact, and in doing so, a helmet —in effect— commits suicide.

In the early days of hard helmets (after leather aviator caps) the idea was to build a helmet strong enough to repel an impact. This worked well for the helmet, but it ignored Newton's First Law of Motion (a.k.a. The Law of Inertia):

> *An object in a state of uniform motion tends to remain in that state of motion, unless acted upon by an external force.*

To understand what this means to our head, let's take a closer look at the inside of it. Our brain rests within our brainpan (skull) and is cushioned by *cerebrospinal fluid* (CSF), which continually flows around our brain and our spine. CSF is vital for many reasons, not the least of which is it stops the brain from slamming into the inside of our skull in the event of a minor fall, or a minor blow to the head.

Cerebrospinal Fluid (CSF) surrounds the brain and protects it from direct contact with the skull.

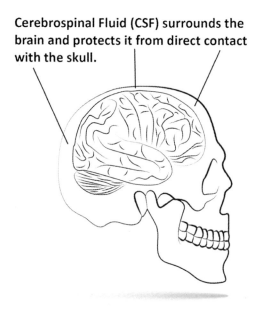

With those early hard-shell helmets, when a rider's head hit the ground (or other object) another physical law came into play: the law of conservation of energy. This law states that energy cannot be destroyed. It can change form, such as when the energy contained in gasoline is converted to mechanical movement, but it cannot be destroyed. Those early shells were built to resist impact —meaning they didn't flex.

A modern helmet protects by —in effect— committing suicide.

Instead they transferred (conserved) the force directly to the rider's skull as absorption liners did not exist.

Let's say that unfortunate rider is traveling a modest 45 miles per hour. Remember, every part of his body was traveling 45 mph, including his brain that is cushioned by CSF. As the shell receives the blow, it transfers the force of it to his skull, abruptly stopping it from moving forward. However, that gelatinous mass that is the brain does not stop; it kept moving forward at 45 mph —remember, The Law of Inertia— and in doing so compresses and overcomes any cushioning effect of the CSF, and slams into the inside of his skull. The shell was designed to survive this hit but, depending upon the amount of force, the rider could count on, at least, a headache or, at worst, the jellification of his brain. Yeah, that's as bad as it sounds.

Surviving the Blow

In 1953 a Professor C.F. Lombard of the University of Southern California developed a helmet with an internal layer designed to buffer and reduce the force of the impact before it reaches the skull. This layer was made from expanded polystyrene (EPS), a closed-cell thermoplastic that can be found in coffee cups, packing material and —still today— helmet liners. Professor Lombard's efforts were funded by the U.S. Navy, and were focused on military use and not motorcycle riders. The application of EPS to motorcycle helmets was left to various helmet manufacturers beginning in the mid-1950s.

Here is a simple review of what a modern helmet does to protect your noggin, in the event you have an unplanned meeting with the ground. As your head slams onto the pavement, the shell bends inward, distributing the force of the blow over a wide area of the shell. This is the helmet's first effort at dissipating the blow. Next, the shell presses in on the EPS liner causing it —the liner— to compress, further lessening the force. If the initial impact is not too great, and the shell and liner do their jobs, the force that reaches your skull will certainly be enough to get your attention, but you'll survive.

Yes, Helmets Do Need to be Replaced Periodically

Every reputable expert will tell you to replace your helmet once it's taken a significant hit. If the shell is visibly fractured, then replacement is obvious. Less obvious is a dented EPS liner. This happens when the shell takes a hit, bends in and compresses the liner, but then the shell returns to its original shape. The problem is the EPS liner remains compressed, rendering it useless if struck again. Don't take a chance —replace the helmet. The replacement period can vary between manufacturers, but I'd suggest replacement every two to three years. And here's a variable you should consider: petroleum fumes (gas, parts cleaner, etc.) can degrade EPS. Don't store your helmet adjacent any such items. In fact, keep your helmet in the house, not the garage.

The original hard helmet shells were made from a variety of materials, including shellacked canvas and pith, a corklike, soft plant tissue. These evolved into the primary shell materials found on today's helmets: fiberglass and thermoplastic and, at the expensive end of things, carbon fiber and Kevlar.

In the early 1970's I owned a motorcycle parts and accessories biz (Trackside) in Northern California. We sold Bell helmets almost exclusively, with the top product going for about a hundred bucks. During this period cheap thermoplastic helmets began to appear on the market. As I recall, $19.99 was a popular price, and they could usually be found in auto parts stores. I refused to sell them as the technology was in its infancy, with the result being these helmets had a tendency to shatter on impact. That shattering did serve to help dissipate force, but it also produced dangerous shards that, in one instance I'm very familiar with, killed the rider. Plastics science has come a long ways since then, and today I have no issue with wearing a helmet made from thermoplastic.

Where Is the Hit Taken?

In 1981 Dietmar Otte of the Medical University Hannover (Germany) released a report on (in part) the distribution of impacts on motorcycle helmets involved in accidents. He evaluated 679 motorcycle accidents, involving 802 riders or passengers protected by helmets. Of the 802 helmets, 598 of them were of a full-face design, which the report refers to as "integral."

At this point, there might be a red flag waving in your mind that raises the question, "Just how relevant is a 30-plus year-old study to today's riders?" In a word, very. It is as relevant as it was 30-plus years ago. Certainly motorcycles have significantly improved over the decades, training has made most riders more proficient than those of years back, and helmet technology has advanced significantly. However, two factors have not changed, 1) The human head is still its fragile self and, 2) riders are still throwing themselves off motorcycles with distressing regularity.

Otte's report is involved and full of numbers and percentages, but when you plot out the impact percentages on an actual helmet one fact becomes crystal clear: two-thirds of the impacts were taken by the front of the helmet. Furthermore, more than one-third of the impacts were located on the chin area alone.

Of the three primary styles of helmets available —Half, Three-Quarter, and Full-Face (so-named for the approximate amount of your head that they cover) — only the full-face style protects your chin; that part of your head that Otte's study showed received more than one-third of the impacts studied. If your preference is for a helmet type other than full-face, I urge you to look closely at Otte's results.

What's Your Excuse?

Over the years, the three most common excuses I've heard for not wearing a full-face helmet are, 1) they restrict peripheral vision, 2) they are too hot in the summer and, 3) you can't hear. Let's look at these a little closer.

The National Highway Traffic Safety Administration mandates that all motorcycle helmets legally sold in the U.S. must have a minimum of 210 degrees of peripheral vision, 105 degrees per side. Human beings …that be us… can see approximately 90 degrees to either side. These numbers show that any legal helmet, full-face or not, will provide sufficient side-to-side vision; more side-to-side vision than you could ever physically use with peripheral vision, in fact. So, why does this vision issue come up every so often?

I think there are two reasons for this. The first is a degree of claustrophobia. I've come across several riders over the years that cannot tolerate being enclosed in a full-face helmet. In the words of one, "I feel like the world is closing in on me." Since the rider already feels claustrophobic in the enclosed helmet, the addition of a chin bar can give the impres-

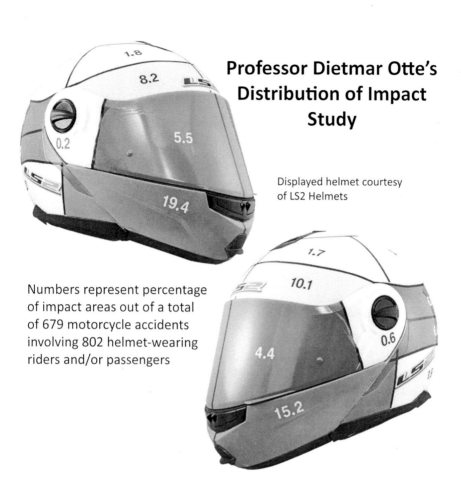

Professor Dietmar Otte's Distribution of Impact Study

Displayed helmet courtesy of LS2 Helmets

Numbers represent percentage of impact areas out of a total of 679 motorcycle accidents involving 802 helmet-wearing riders and/or passengers

Distribution of Impact
    Front:

Chin	34.6%	
Eyeport	9.9%	
Forehead	18.3%	
Upper Forehead	3.5%	

TOTAL IMPACT % TO FRONT OF HELMET   **66.3%**
     Sides, Rear, Top   **33.3%**

Two-thirds of the impacts were taken at the front of the helmet.

sion to some that the width of the eye port (that 210 degrees) has been reduced. Legally, this cannot be the case.

The second issue is improper fit. If the helmet does not fit snugly and properly on your head, there is the possibility that it is sitting too far forward, and this would reduce the effective peripheral vision. Ill-fitting helmets are not unusual, just look around the next time you're with a group of riders. While, again, adding that full-face chin bar brings more attention to the side views. Fixing this issue can be as simple as wearing a helmet that fits properly.

> ## The top three reasons mentioned for not wearing a full-face helmet:
> 1. They restrict vision
> 2. They can be too hot
> 3. You can't hear
>
> **Two-and-a-half of these reasons are incorrect. What about the remaining half?**
> **Yes, they *can* get hot in very hot weather.**

The second popular excuse is that full-face helmets are "too hot in the summer." Yes, they can be hotter than an open-face helmet, particularly in slow traffic —but, interestingly, out on the highway, a full-face can actually be cooler to wear as it blocks the direct heat blast to your face. I've worn a full-face for more than 40 years, in all types of weather and conditions. The heat issue has never caused me a problem.

And then there's the "I can't hear well in a full-face helmet" excuse. I've yet to find any evidence that a full-face helmet blocks any more sound than an open-face. There is a widespread perception that you cannot hear as well in a full-face helmet but lacking credible evidence this will remain just a perception.

Helmet Safety Standards

The British were the first to take a serious look at the design and testing of motorcycle helmets, beginning in the 1940s. In 1952, this work resulted in the world's first formalized motorcycle helmet standard, the British Standard 1868: Crash Helmets for Racing Motor Cyclists. The significant difference with this standard, compared to previous efforts, is that in addition to outlining how a helmet should be built, it also defined how a helmet should be tested.

Differing Helmet Standards

Throughout the world, there are dozens of different standards that a helmet must meet in order to be legally sold as a motorcycle helmet. In the U.S. the three most familiar standards are:

- Snell
- DOT
- ECE

There are helmets on the market that do not meet any of the legal standards. These are referred to as "novelty helmets" or, more correctly, "crap." In my opinion, manufacturers and distributors of these are guilty of criminal negligence. They are knowingly offering a product that does not meet minimal safety standards, and are doing it to circumvent the law. Furthermore, these helmets can offer a very false sense of security to an uninformed rider.

• Snell

In 1959, the Snell Memorial Foundation published the first U.S. construction and testing standards for helmets used in car racing. Developed by Dr. George Snively, these standards were an outgrowth of an investigation into the death of William "Pete" Snell during an amateur sports car racing accident in1956. Since 1959, the Snell certification of helmets has expanded to include usage by motorcycle and bicycle riders, among others.

In order to qualify for Snell certification, a helmet manufacturer's products must meet the testing standards issued by Snell and helmets must be submitted for testing. Beginning in 1970, these standards have been revised every five years.

• DOT

To be legally sold as a motorcycle helmet in the U.S., a manufacturer's products must meet federal standards as determined by the Department of Transportation (DOT), as laid out in their Federal Motor Vehicle Safety Standard (FMVSS) 218. This standard was implemented in 1974 and addresses (as do the other standards) a helmet's inner liner thickness, chinstrap, and weight. The DOT standard does not concern itself with helmet style as all styles can be found with DOT approval stickers. And just so you understand, regardless of any other standard a helmet might carry, it still must meet the DOT requirements in order to be sold in this country.

The biggest, and off-cited problem with the DOT standard is that it is based upon the honor system, as the Fed relies on the manufacturer's word that their helmets are in compliance with FMVSS 218; they do not test the helmets like Snell does. The Department of Transportation can, however, demand that the manufacturer provide test results. Additionally, The National Highway Traffic Safety Administration (NHTSA), the enforcement arm of the DOT, is authorized to obtain and test random helmet samples. Companies that manufacture, sell, and/or deliver non-compliant helmets are subject to fines up to $5,000 per violation.

The only mandatory aspect of the DOT standard is that the DOT sticker be affixed to helmets that the manufacturers claim meet FM-VSS 218 requirements. Several years ago it was easy to find fake DOT compliance stickers on novelty helmets. Fortunately this bit of fraud has subsided. Unfortunately, novelty helmets continue to be produced, sold, and worn.

• ECE

Though relatively new in the U.S., the ECE R22-05 standard is the most prevalent helmet standard in the world. Developed by UNECE (United Nations Economic Commission for Europe), it was first published in 1995. One of the significant differences with the ECE standard is that it requires the manufacturer to submit a batch of helmets (up to 50) for testing, in advance of production. Additionally, the manufacturer must submit to verification of its quality procedures during production.

Interesting, but just where does this leave us, the riders? It seems that "confused," more often than not, might be the answer to that. Let me clarify a few things. First off, regardless of the helmet rating, there is no guarantee of protection level. While this might seems obvious, some riders tend to believe that wearing a helmet makes them impervious to injury.

Secondly, regardless of the helmet's rating, unless it fits properly you are not being protected as well as you could be. If you are unsure how a helmet should fit, talk with the expert at the dealership you frequent.

Thirdly, it's reasonable to ask, "Which helmet standard will provide the maximum protection?"

That answer is tied up in never-ending arguments so, lacking a consensus among experts, let me toss in my opinion. If you carefully read each of the testing standards, it's possible to reach a conclusion that says the Snell standard favors impact resistance, while the DOT and ECE standards favor impact absorption. My personal preference favors the absorption of impact, but I have worn Snell helmets for almost 50 years.

Every credible professional motorcycle (and car) racing organization in the U.S. approves Snell- and ECE-rated helmets for competition use. They do

There are helmets on the market that do not meet any of the legal standards. These are referred to as "novelty helmets" or, more correctly, "crap."

not approve DOT-only helmets. I will not wear a DOT-only helmet. Not because I don't trust the government standard but, rather, because of the absence of regular, periodic —rather than random— objective testing.

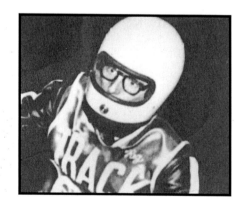

In the 60's I raced with one of the original Bell "Star" helmets. I'm wearing "safety glasses" here because the eyeport shield, which slid into grooves in the rubber grommet, had turned a sickly yellow from contact with the rubber.

Hearing Protection

Ideally, hearing protection should start before any non-age-related hearing loss takes place. Many of us riders don't think much about protecting our hearing until we notice a loss and/or our doctor raises the issue. Once you've lost your hearing it is not something you can get back through diet or exercise. You have to resort to hearing aids that are an expensive solution, and they will only improve your hearing, not restore it completely. The solution is to be proactive, and that simply means wear earplugs when you ride.

Noise Reduction Ratings

Before I get to the pros and cons of each earplug type, let's review a misunderstood subject: Noise Reduction Ratings (NRR). Quality earplugs must meet federal standards as determined by the Occupational Safety & Health Administration (OSHA), and be tested and approved by the American National Standards Institute (ANSI). The result of this testing is a noise reduction decibel rating. This rating will tell you just how much noise it will block... if you understand it.

For example, the highest NRR rating approved by OSHA is "NRR33." This implies that the use of these earplugs will reduce noise to your eardrum by 33 db, right? Uh... they won't. What it actually means is that under controlled conditions in the ANSI lab, a 100 db sound would be reduced to 67 db, which is a 33 db reduction under perfect conditions.

ANSI recognizes that perfect conditions do not exist in the real world. Each of us has slightly different shaped ear canals, and we don't all insert the earplug properly, so they've calculated a formula to determine the actual noise reduction: (NRR db – 7)/2.

Let's say you're using NRR33 earplugs, and riding a motorcycle

The highest Noise Reduction Rating approved by OSHA is 33 dB

with a 100 db exhaust sound level. Applying that formula would make your real-world noise reduction (33-7)/2 =13. Now, subtract that 13 from the 100 db sound, and you see that the noise level is knocked down to 87 db, not the assumed 67 db. This begs the question: Why don't they just label them as NRR13 to begin with? Just another one of those great mysteries of life, I guess.

Three Types of Earplugs for Riders

For motorcycle riding, there are three primary types of earplugs. Unless you have specific reasons not to, always use earplugs with the highest NRR number, which is usually 32 or 33.

1. Wax/Cotton

I only mention them so that you know not to use them. Their primary use is for sleeping or, for example, while flying. There are a couple reasons why I don't recommend using this type of earplug. For one, they are made from wax, with cotton threads to help hold them together and they usually need to be softened up before they can be inserted in the ear. This can make these earplugs difficult to insert in colder weather. Once in your ear, these earplugs firm up, but this can cause problems as any jaw movement will break the seal with your ear canal and let noise intrude. Another issue is that they are not very sanitary, as they pick up dust, earwax, and hair. Additionally, they don't generally have an NRR number. Don't bother with these.

2. Foam

The best foam earplugs are made from a polyurethane variant often referred to as "memory foam" for its ability to return to its original shape after being compressed. They are available in a wide variety of NRR ratings. They are reusable, but will collect dirt in short order.

3. Custom-Molded Silicone

If you frequent motorcycle events you've probably seen a vendor inserting liquid silicone into a rider's ears. What first looks like a medieval torture of sorts is actually a fitting for custom-molded earplugs. The idea is that, since everyone's ear canal is slightly different, to be most effective the earplugs should be custom made.

You can also purchase kits and mold your own earplugs. Notable with some of these kits is that they do offer an NRR rating, with the highest I've seen being NRR26.

Molded earplugs sound good in theory, and there are certainly riders that high-five the idea. I'm not one of them. In my experience, these molded plugs tend to cause heat build-up in my ear canals to the point where I have to pull them out; I find them very uncomfortable. Additionally, as they are not as pliable as foam plugs, they don't readily accommodate the normal narrowing of the ear canal during a hot ride. Also, because each custom set is unique, there is no NRR rating (except as noted above) although the various vendors I've spoken with claim a "high rating." If you believe molded plugs are the way to go, I suggest you have them made by a licensed audiologist. They will work with you to determine the optimum material used and will be able to give you an NRR number.

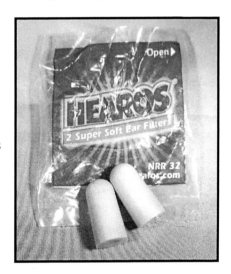

Unless you have special and unusual needs, properly used foam earplugs should work as well as anything, including molded plugs, and are significantly less expensive. In particular, I like the Hearos brand. For around five bucks you can buy enough foam plugs to last all riding season. This is about one-tenth of what custom-molded plugs will cost you.

Sunglasses

Sunglasses are an obvious accessory for riders but many don't understand why you should wear them, other than to cut the sun's harsh, bright light. Certainly that's a good reason, but an even better one is that they can protect your eyes from ultraviolet rays.

We are continually being bombarded by the sun's radiation, with most of it hitting us as visible light. A small portion of this radiation, however, arrives in the form of ultraviolet light (UV) rays, so called because the wavelength of this light (as with sound, light travels in waves) is very short and just beyond the wavelength of the color violet. Thus, ultraviolet.

By nature, the shorter radiation waves are, the more energy they contain. This high energy can cause damage to our body's tissue down to the cellular level. The most visible impact of the damage is sunburn and, in extreme cases, skin cancer. Less visible, but highly dangerous is the damage that can be caused to the sensitive and vulnerable construction of our eyes. For instance, UV radiation has been cited as a factor that can lead to age-related macular degeneration (AMD), as discussed in Chapter 4.

There are three different wavelengths of UV radiation: UV-A, UV-B, and UV-C. Only UV-A and UV-B rays actually reach the surface of the earth; they are the ones we need to protect ourselves from. We do this — if we're smart — by using sunscreen and wearing protective clothing like hats, long-sleeved shirts and sunglasses.

So what kind of sunglasses do we need? Well, spending many hundreds of dollars on sunglasses can buy us big-name style and exclusivity, but not necessarily improved protection. Whatever the price tag, we need to make sure our sunglasses protect us first and foremost from UV-A and UV-B radiation. We also want to make sure our sunglasses have a high-impact distortion-free

...spending many hundreds of dollars on sunglasses can buy us big-name style and exclusivity, but not necessarily improved protection.

lens, and are able to shield our eyes from wind and dust. Yes, your $300 puttin'-on-the-Ritz sunglasses can do this, but you can also spend a tenth, or less, of that and get equal protection.

A company called Ztek makes my riding sunglasses of choice. I discovered them at the BMW dealer in Daytona several years ago. They are reasonably stylish, meet all my safety requirements, have proven to be tough and scratch resistant, and cost me all of $12. The secret here is that they are "safety glasses" generally sold in hardware stores, rather than trendy boutiques. I carry three pair; clear, yellow, and tinted. (Yes, a clear lens can still protect you from UV-A and UV-B rays.)

Polarized Sunglasses

We all know that having polarized lens sunglasses is a good thing, right? Well, yes… and no. Polarization is excellent at cutting glare, but if you are wearing polarized sunglasses and looking through a polarized face shield you'll see what is known as an interference pattern or, more technically, a moiré pattern. Put another way, it can approximate what you may or may not have seen when you were "herbed up" back in the 60's… a slightly out of focus, prismatic view. Certainly an entertaining sight if you're sitting in a bean bag chair, but not so safe if you're riding a motorcycle.

To understand how polarized sunglasses through a polarized face shield can create moiré, we need to briefly understand how light and polarized sunglasses work. Glare happens because sunlight, when reflected off of shiny surfaces, reflects back in the same plane as the surface. That is, it strikes a flat, horizontal surface and the light is reflected back horizontally, which makes it polarized light. This polarized reflection then hits your eyes as a bright glare. To counteract this polarization, polarized sunglasses have a very thin layer of microscopically narrow vertical stripes applied to the sunglass lens. This vertical orientation of the stripes breaks up the horizontal reflection, thereby dramatically reducing glare. And yes, we do see some vertically polarized light, but the majority of glare comes from horizontal surfaces such as roadways, bodies of water, snow, and those beautifully chromed mufflers. When you wear polarized sunglasses behind a polarized face shield you are looking through two layers of vertical stripes. As you move your head — even slightly — those two layers merge and diverge, causing the annoying, not-so-groovy interference pattern (moiré). I enjoy the benefits of a polarized lens, but I prefer to use it on my face shield, not my riding sunglasses. (Unless I'm sitting in a bean bag chair. Then I can wear both.)

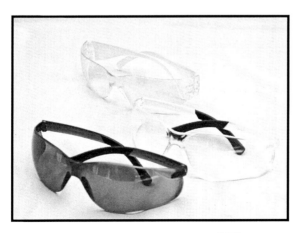

Ztek Glasses
Take my word for it, there are tinted, clear, and orange versions shown here. If you buy direct, the cost can be less than $3 each!

Staying Warm With Heated Clothes

I'll be the first to admit that I'm a certified wimp when it comes to cold weather: I don't like it, never have. Here in Santa Cruz our winters would hardly register compared to those in the more northern regions of our country. We get a lot of temps in the 40s and mornings can see it dip into the 30s, but snow, ice and sleet mercifully stay away except on rare occasions. Rain however, can be significant with around 60 inches being the winter norm.

As mild as some might consider these conditions, I can usually find reason to whine about the cold, particularly when I travel. There are numerous reasons why the cold affects people differently. For some, it's a medical condition like anemia or hypothyroidism that heightens cold sensitivity, for others

I'll be the first to admit that I'm a certified wimp when it comes to cold weather.

it is a lack of insulating fat, and for others it can be degraded circulatory function that creates a diminished blood flow to extremities (common in elderly people who often get cold hands and feet).

A good solution to this cold problem is heated clothing. Personally, I use a heated jacket liner and heated gloves, but heated socks, pants, vests, and bibs are also available. If this is the route you want to take, you have a couple of decisions to make. First, do you want to power up this gear with batteries, or connect to your motorcycle's electrical system? Battery power simplifies things as you don't need the connection to your motorcycle, but I've found they do not get as warm as a connected system, and you're always having to carry and change batteries. The life expectancy of the batteries is usually only a couple of hours, and the power output is about half that of connected systems. The newest in consumer battery tech — lithium-ion batteries — have a significantly higher power output and longer life, but they are also more expensive.

Getting Connected

Connected systems require a 12-volt outlet on your motorcycle. This can be either the familiar "cigarette socket," a BMW-style outlet, or the basic SAE polarized plug. Most motorcycles now come equipped with outlets. In the case of my Triumph Tiger it has one adjacent the triple clamp, and another under the seat. This is a common layout for

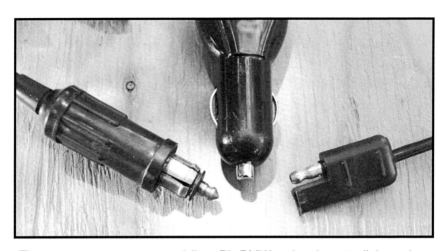

Three ways to get connected (L to R): BMW-style, cigarette lighter plug, and polarized SAE. If you have one, but need the other, adapters are available

adventure motorcycles. If your motorcycle does not come equipped with a 12-volt outlet, they are readily available and can be mounted to any motorcycle.

Regardless of the connector you use make sure it has a waterproof cover that protects the fitting when your heated clothing (or any other 12 volt accessory) is not connected, and that there is a fuse between the battery and the connector tip. Do not, by the way, connect any device directly to the battery without a fuse in the line. Additionally, I recommend that you coat the metal-to-metal parts of the connectors with an anti-corrosive paste. Any corrosion on an electrical connector acts as resistance, with the result being less of the 12 volts you need getting to your heated clothing.

Regulating the Heat

Your heated clothing itself plugs into a controller that functions as a thermostat and allows you to regulate the temperature. And this is where you'll have another decision to make: a single or dual temperature controller. Both are sold as additional-cost accessories. If you are buying a single heated item — for example gloves or a liner — a basic, single-knob controller works just fine. If, however, you purchase a jacket liner and a pair of gloves, you should buy the dual controller. While you can use a single controller, it really doesn't work satisfactorily as you will have to set the same temperature for both items. In practice what this means is that you'll have to choose between the liner being the right temperature and the gloves too hot or cold, or vice versa. The dual controller eliminates this problem by allowing you to set each garment's temperature individually.

Controllers generally come with one of the three connectors mentioned above. Do not connect the controller directly to your battery; plug it into the outlet on your motorcycle.

Finally, if you're looking to keep your body warm electrically you'll have to decide just how much heat you need. If you ride in a very cold climate, or like to stay on the toasty side wherever you ride,

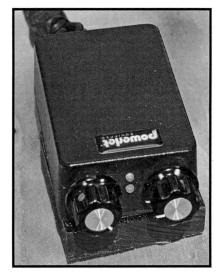

A dual controller allows you to set different temperatures for different garments.

you can buy electrified gloves, socks, pants, vest, jacket liner and neck warmer. In my case, I opted for just the liner and gloves. This combination has served me well in all but the very coldest conditions.

12.

There is a delicate ridge one must ride between
fear and reason on a motorcycle—lean too far
in either direction and there will be consequences.

Lily Brooks-Dalton

School Days

During the early years of this century, track schools and track days sprouted up like weeds at a foreclosed home. Motorcycle sales were booming, racing was in full swing, and the serious sportbike riders, in particular, were beginning to realize that, "Hey, maybe I ought to get a bit of training on how to properly ride this thing!" Track schools had been around for a number of years, notably Keith Code's "California Superbike School," and Reg Pridmore's "CLASS," but most riders considered these race-oriented schools and — as street riders —schools that didn't apply to them. Also, more than a few of the track schools (not the aforementioned) made no pretense towards being anything other than an excuse to ride on a racetrack. As the number of schools increased, so did the competition and the demand that these schools begin to appeal to a wider audience. That is when we began to see an increase in pure street bikes in schools — cruisers, touring bikes, etc. — and more emphasis on teaching street skills. The pioneer in street-oriented schools is Streetmasters Motorcycle Workshops. If you've taken a school or two, you likely know their worth. If you haven't, let me lay out some reasons why you should do so.

Experience vs. Competence

There is the tendency to equate experience with competence. Unfortunately, "the longer you do something, the better you must be at doing it" is not necessarily true. In fact, I might go so far as to say that the mere act of doing something for years can actually make you less competent. Without proper instruction, most of us will simply continue to repeat and reinforce our bad habits year after year. One of the most obvious examples of this involves braking a motorcycle. Proper training shows the importance of using the front brake, regardless of motorcycle type. Yet, it is very easy to spot riders who use the rear brake exclusively, and will defend to their death —in some cases, literally— the right to ignore the front brake.

The root cause of many riding problems with older riders is that we were largely self-taught or taught by a friend or relative. That informal training method usually began with a lot of falling down until, with practice, we were able to acquire the basic skills that kept the rubber side down and between the lines. Most of us taught this way usually become decent enough riders, however, any bad habits picked up during the learning phase have a tendency to stick around until someone shows us otherwise.

I took my first track school at the age of 49. With more than 25 years of riding under my belt I figured there wasn't a lot that I was going to learn. By the end of that humbling day it was crystal clear to me, and the instructors, that I really didn't have more than 25 years experience. What I had was one year's experience that I'd repeated more than 25 times.

The root cause of many riding problems with older riders is that we were largely self-taught.

The most significant aspect of track school education is the many pairs of expert eyes that watch and evaluate you. With the better schools, the day consists of alternating classroom and track sessions. The classes explain the dynamics of riding, outline the track exercises, and answer any questions you might have. Out on the track you put the exercises to work, and are closely monitored by the instructors.

Track Skills Benefit the Street Rider

One of the excuses used by riders for not attending a school is that they have no desire to roadrace; they just want to enjoy the street. That may be true, but the skills learned on that track are largely transferable to the street. Additionally, as the training takes placed in a closed environment with no oncoming traffic, track schools give you the opportunity to concentrate on learning, rather than having to deal with the distractions of the street. The responsible schools segregate riders according to their experience and abilities, and set firm speed and passing rules.

The biggest benefit of track schools is that they instill confidence. One of the misunderstandings about schools is that they teach you to go fast. No, they don't. What they teach is smoothness. While most riders discover that they are lapping the track quicker by the end of the class, it's not because that is the intent of the school. Rather, it's because they have learned how to ride smoother and with far less nervousness and drama.

At the end of your first track school several things will be apparent. Most importantly, you'll realize that there is a lot more to being a competent rider than you realized. (And that you are *less* competent than you thought.)

Selecting a School

There are dozens of good track schools spread about the country. That does not mean, however, that every one meets your needs. Though similar, each is different, and it is this nuanced difference that you need to understand before you plunk down the significant amount of money required to attend one.

Your first step in selecting a school is to understand what you want to get out of it. Are you looking to improve your all-around street skills, or is becoming a track day regular or a roadracer your goal? If you are undecided about this, I suggest you approach the schools with the idea of improving your street skills because if your street skills are below par, jumping onto a racing motorcycle is not the smartest of first steps. Another reason for doing it this way is to familiarize yourself with a racetrack. The track environment is quite different from that of the street, but many riders don't realize just how different it is until they are actually on one, at which time more than a few have decided, uh… this isn't for me.

Track day or track school? There is a big difference; Choose wisely.

Let's back up here and repeat things a bit as your safety will depend upon it.

When researching rider training, you'll see two offerings come up: track days and track schools; these are two totally different things. A track day puts you and your motorcycle on a racetrack. The organizers check your motorcycle for overall good condition, see that your tires are sufficiently new and up to proper pressure, and look over your approved full-face helmet and full riding gear.

While the organizers will monitor your time on the track, you will not be given any instructions and, generally won't hear anything from the

the organizers unless you are overly squidish, or really screwing up. The better schools will slot you into a group with similar experience. Then, it's just you, the track, and any number of other riders who want to show how fast they are. It can be an intimidating first-time experience.

I strongly suggest that you do not sign up for a track day until you've attended a track school. A credible track school is a tightly controlled environment that does everything it can to assure that you belong on a track,

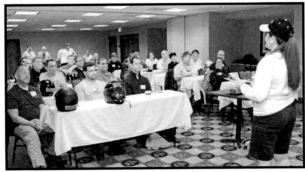

Classroom instruction is a critical component of the best training schools. Here, Streetmaster's Nancy Foote discusses the plan for the day. Photo by Bruce Laidlaw

you are riding only with those of similar skill, and that you receive the necessary instruction in order to improve and refine your riding skills. Think of it this way: at a track day you may, or may not, improve your

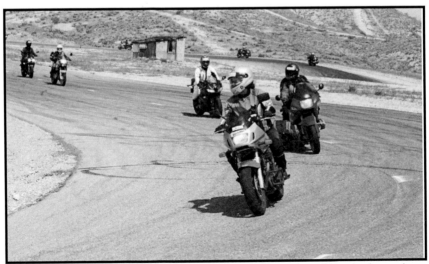

Out on the track you are closely monitored. Note the white dash marks down the track's center. Streetmasters uses these to assure that the training matches what you'll find on the street. Photo by Bruce Laidlaw

skills independently; at a track school you improve your skills with guidance from a number of experts.

Putting your wheels on a racetrack can be a very fun, exhilarating experience that every rider — regardless of what they ride — should have. It can also be a dangerous, painful and expensive experience if not approached the right way. The difference between the two depends upon the decisions you make up front. Put your ego aside, then think about your skill level and experience, and then choose the school that fits you best. How much you learn and how safe you'll be is largely based on these decisions that you make before arriving at the track.

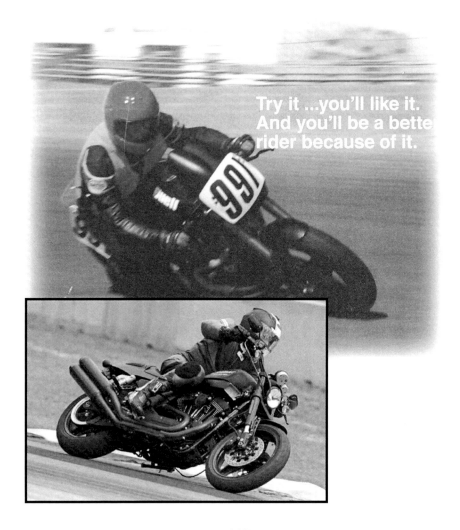

Try it ...you'll like it. And you'll be a better rider because of it.

13.

Yeah, I'm 72, but that's just 22 celsius
Arké

On the Road

Want a more enjoyable ride? Being physically and mentally fit before you climb onto the saddle will help increase comfort and longevity, but there are also a number of things you can do during your ride to make your long treks more enjoyable.

A good part of my riding over the years has been as a function of my journalistic efforts, whether it be evaluating motorcycles, heading to events, or logging miles to write travel articles. This "work" created a bad riding habit: I was always in too much of a hurry chasing tight schedules and deadlines to really appreciate the ride itself. This dawned on me several years ago as I was riding up the Oregon coast searching out lighthouses for an article. This tour took me down several interesting roads I wouldn't have otherwise taken in my previous life of deadlines and schedules; I would have raced right past them.

"So, my first bit of travel advice is to not forget the roses."

So, my first bit of travel advice is to not forget the roses. You know, the ones you are supposed to stop and smell along the way. Slow your schedule down. You won't travel the same number of miles, but you'll better enjoy the miles you do travel. For most, this situation usually pops up with your annual vacation. You have two weeks and you're gonna cram in as much travel as possible!

Dawn-to-dusk saddle time might impress the Iron Butt folks, but it puts the rest of us at risk. As we tire our reflexes slow and our thinking gets a bit mushy. Neither condition is conducive to a safe ride. Besides, what's more interesting: telling someone how many miles you traveled in a day (as they feign interest) or describing the interesting sights you saw after taking a back-roads ride?

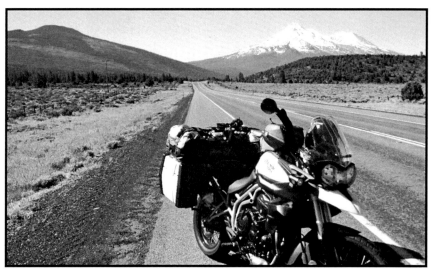

Sometimes the best part of a motorcycle trip is stopping to look back at where you've been. In this case, it's Mt. Shasta, California.

Asleep at the Bars

Apparently, none of us get enough sleep. According to the Center for Disease Control (CDC), a study taken in 2009 indicates that "insufficient sleep is a public health epidemic." The study strongly suggests this "… may be caused by broad scale societal factors such as round-the-clock access to technology and work schedules… ." As we age, we have a tendency to sleep less — not because we don't need it, but because the various effects of a longer life such as a bad back or painful hips keep us from getting a proper amount of rest. I'm guessing this really isn't news to you, but what you might not clearly understand is its effect on your motorcycle riding. This sleep deprivation has two primary negative effects which require our attention: physical fatigue and mental fatigue.

When we are physically fatigued we are unable to function normally. We are physically weaker, and incapable of reacting as quickly as we would were we rested. Mental fatigue shows up first as drowsiness; the "I can't keep my eyes open" feeling. Medicos refer to this as "somnolence."

Not surprisingly, mental fatigue slows your processing of information as well as the required reaction to it. This is where it really begins to affect your riding. Safely riding a motorcycle requires a constant processing of information; much more processing than when driving a car. For me, mental fatigue often manifests itself into a thousand-yard-stare condition wherein my eyes are set on the horizon, but my mind has clicked on the pause button. Mental fatigue almost always arrives hand-in-hand with physical fatigue brought on by too many hours in the saddle.

An example: A few years back I was on Highway 70 west of Glenwood Springs, Colorado. This is a good motorcycle road (for an interstate) bordered by the Colorado River. I leaned into a turn and immediately found a large metal jack handle directly in my path. A quick bar flick got me safely around it. Had I been fatigued or zoned out I might not have been able to react as quickly, with the result not being pretty.

Remember that the idea behind vacations is to rest while enjoying yourself. Also remember that by the time that annual respite rolls around, most of us are sorely in need of rest and relaxation. All too often we plan our trips, pack carefully, and sleep fitfully the night before we leave, only to kick-off the next morning what feels like an all-out endurance haul toward a motel reservation a few hundred miles down the road. This race to the motel often controls where, how often, and for how long we stop along the way. Then, once we're at our destination what follows is usually a large

...by the end of our vacation... we wish we could take a vacation.

dinner, maybe a drink or two, and often a late night followed by another early morning where we rinse and repeat the same routine. Is it any wonder that by the end of our vacation... we wish we could take a vacation.

Why keep repeating the same old exhausting routine? Why would we want to sacrifice the quality of our ride for boring mileage quantity? Remember this next time you're planning to spend six days of your seven-day vacation in the saddle blowing past all the sights you could be seeing.

When the Body Needs Sleep, It Sleeps

Over the years I've entered several 1,000 mile/24 hour events. As the name implies these are simple events that require you to do nothing more than ride a minimum of 1,000 miles in that allotted time. I can't say that I've found them enjoyable because they can be grueling. I guess more than anything else it's the challenge that brings me to the starting line. Simple math shows that you need only average a tick under 42 miles per hour to meet the goal. Sounds simple enough, but there's usually a generous portion of the route where it's difficult to hit that average, and it is very difficult to ride continually for 24 hours. The key is to "put time in the bank." That is, make up time where the route allows higher speeds. Also, you need to budget time for food/gas/pee stops and a catnap or three.

The first one of these that I entered was in the late 80s in Northern California. The event was scheduled from midnight to midnight. The experienced riders knew to adjust their sleeping schedule several days in advance of the event. My strategy was to grab a nap in the afternoon before the start... my first wrong step in an adventure with sleep deprivation.

The first several hundred miles had me thinking this was a piece-o-cake; superslab all the way from Livermore to Redding. At Redding we struck off on Highway 299 —a great, winding motorcycle road when the sun is up and you're rested. Neither condition was present. By midmorning I was beginning to see animals that weren't there, and my mind

The next I remember is waking up. No, I hadn't crashed.

began wandering off on its own. I recall passing through Happy Camp on Highway 96. The next I remember is waking up. No, I hadn't crashed. In fact, my Harley FXR was safely parked by the side of the road, and I was sitting on the ground on the bike's upside, leaning against the motor. I couldn't recall having stopped, any part of my nap, or any pain from the burn on my jacket from leaning against the hot motor. That episode taught me that I need to schedule my naps before — not during — the event.

In 2006 I learned another lesson about sleep deprivation. I entered a 24-hour sportbike event that traversed a wide range of Southern California real estate. On my way to the start in SoCal, I got sick. It wasn't a big deal, and it passed within a few hours. After checking in at the

"As I had turned this into a bit of a personal race, adrenaline kept me moving and focused.

host motel I left a message with the desk for a 4:30 a.m. wake-up call, and headed for the sack. Still a bit woozy, I wanted to log as many sleep hours as possible before the start. The event start was staggered between 5 a.m. and 6 a.m.

As the gods would have it, the clerk missed my wake-up call. I woke at 5:40 a.m., with 20 minutes to the start deadline. I came to the line with two minutes to spare, and with everyone else long gone. I had a thousand miles in front of me, and a deadline of 5:58 a.m., the next

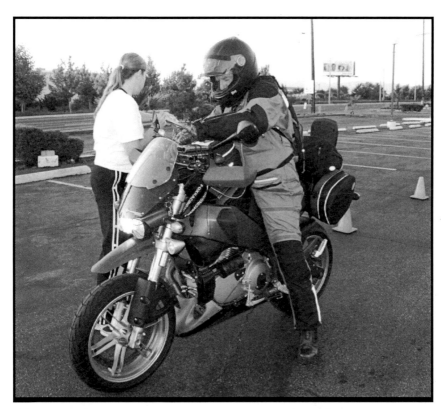

At the start line with two minutes to spare: rested, confident, and ignorant.

morning. I had slept well, and the first half of the ride was in daylight, so I felt confident that everything was under control. This confidence lasted for about 17 hours.

Because of my late start I got it into my head that I was behind schedule. I really wasn't as all of us were on our own schedule. Or maybe it was the ex-racer in me; I couldn't stand the fact that there was anyone in front of me. So instead of just "banking" some time during the day, I made it my mission to pass riders. There were 34 entries, and I did manage to bag about a half-a-dozen of them as they "banked" time.

As I had turned this into a bit of a personal race, adrenaline kept me moving and focused. There's this thing about adrenaline, though... It's like running on nitrous; you go like hell, then you run out and your body says, "OK, that's it. I quit." I hit that point at about 11 o'clock at night.

I was on the Maricopa Highway (Highway 33) having left Frazier Park about an hour before, heading for Ojai. I was tired, but everything was OK. That part of the world is remote, dark, and the moon was busy someplace else. Animals are always a concern on roads such as these, so I lowered my speed. As I rounded a turn the bike began to wobble a bit, but I was able to straighten it out. Next turn, same thing. Something was wrong. My speedometer told the story; I was barely moving fast enough to stay upright. I had no sense of speed. I was, in effect, "sleepriding." It was time to stop. Luckily a short nap refreshed me enough (I carry an alarm clock on these events) to where I could continue, and by some miracle I finished within the allotted time.

What these two incidences showed me is that fatigue can be insidious, and it can sneak up and slap us aside the head before we know it. Fortunately, I learned these lessons without sacrificing life or limb, but it just as easily could have gone the other way.

Your trips may not be of the 1,000/24 kind, but fatigue can affect you just as easily on a normal day trip. Planning your sleep can be just as important as planning your route.

At the finish line: "I will never do this again ... until the next time."

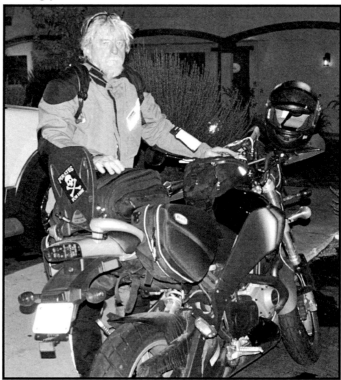

How to Avoid "I Didn't See Him!"

"I didn't see him," is a recurring statement in car vs. motorcycle accident reports. It is usually said in anguish and with high credibility; the driver truly did not see the oncoming motorcycle as they were merging lanes or proceeding through a stop sign.

This statement has bothered me throughout my riding years, and that it is said so often led me to believe there exists something odd about these often-fatal encounters. Can all these accidents be the result of bad drivers or riders, or is there something else at play here? In truth, there are several factors that impact how we see the world. One factor is psychological; oftentimes we see what we expect to see. In this case, non-riding car drivers often do not see motorcycles because they are looking for other cars and don't expect to see motorcycles. The other two factors that come into play are physiological and behavioral, or, physically how our eyes take in and interpret information and how carefully we look at the world around us.

What I've written here is aimed at helping you better understand the physiological and behavioral conditions that affect how well we see and are seen by the world. While we can't change how other people see, the idea is to keep ourselves safe by changing our own observation habits, and with more awareness of how the world sees us.

Physiological Eyesight and the Limitations of Our Eyes

In my research I've learned that the physiological foundation for the "I didn't see him" response goes a long way towards explaining just what happens in those car vs. motorcycle encounters. This physiological aspect also helps to explain what we as riders can do to avoid becoming Victim #1 in an accident report.

How the Eyeball Works

The human eyeball is a complex organ that receives light rays bounced off of reflective surfaces, converts those light rays into electrical impulses, and then sends them — via the optic nerve — to the brain where they are interpreted as images. The answer to our "didn't see him" mystery rests with the manner in which our eyes process these light rays.

Eyesight happens when light passes through the cornea (the eye's transparent front) where it is focused on the pupil that resides in the

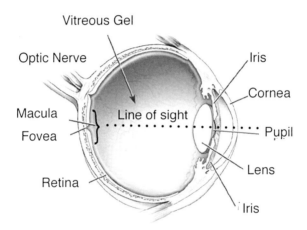

center of the colored iris. In addition to further focusing the light the pupil also controls the amount of light that it allows to pass. This is why our pupils are small (*miotic*) in bright sunlight and large (*dilated*) in the dark. From the pupil the light travels through the lens where it is even more tightly focused before traveling to the retina. And there's where it gets interesting.

The retina is a thin, light-sensitive layer on the interior of the eyeball. It contains millions of photoreceptors that react to varying levels of light and color. There are two primary types of photoreceptors: rods and cones, so named because of their shapes. Rods are very light sensitive, but do not react to color, and are most effective at night. Cones require brighter light before reacting, but do react to color. Cones come into play, primarily, during the daylight hours. The human eye contains more than

125 million rods and cones, with the bulk of them (more than 99 percent) being light-sensitive rods.

Near the center of the retina is the macula, and in its center is the very small fovea centralis (approximately 0.00787 inches wide) that is responsible for generating the visual acuity that allows us to clearly discern details and colors.

Keep that in mind, and then add this: In order to discern the necessary levels of details, *the reflected light from objects must strike the macula and, in particular, the fovea centralis directly, not at an angle.* For that to happen, the object(s) in question must be no more than approximately two degrees (in each direction) off of center. Putting this more simply, in order for us to see something correctly, we must be looking *directly* at it. This is called foveola vision. Let me repeat this, because it's very important: in order to see something correctly, we must be looking directly at it. So, if a motorist is looking at other cars, at pedestrians, at their radios — at anything other than you head-on — chances are good they are not seeing you at all.

In order to see something correctly, we must be looking directly at it.

But what about peripheral vision? When we see things with our peripheral vision they are not head on and, because of this, the reflected light is handled by the rods mostly located outside of the macula. And remember, rods, although light sensitive, do not react to color and do not have the same acuity as cones, so the picture we get from our peripheral vision is a bit blurred and certainly lacks the detail we need. Again: To see something correctly, we must look directly at it. Put another way; do not depend upon peripheral vision to keep you safe.

A Glance Does Not See What Needs Be Seen

There is another aspect to this that contributes to things not being seen: *saccades*. As applied here, a saccade is a quick movement of our eyes. For example, as we read our eyes are making a series of saccades as they see a word, and move along to the next one. While it feels like we are smoothly tracking each line of type, the reality is our eyes are moving in a quick, jerky manner from word to word. The interval between saccades is known as the point of fixation and is the point where we actually see a word. The quicker the glances, the shorter the duration of each point of fixation. In other words, read the sentence quick and your point of fixation jumps quickly creating visual gaps; slow down and the amount of information you take in increases as your eyes are given time to interpret the information received by longer-duration fixation points.

Now, think for a minute about how a four-way stop works, and what happens physically as we look left and right quickly or slowly. As we glance from side to side, our eyes are performing a series of rapid saccades. The quicker the glances, the shorter the duration of the points of fixation. Remember, the only time we actually see something is during those points of fixation; during saccades we are effectively blind. Glance left and right quickly at your four-way stop and you're likely to wiz by

Remember, the only time we actually see something is during those points of fixation; during saccades we are effectively blind.

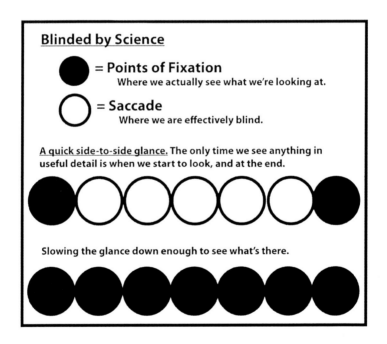

all sorts of details as your eyes leap from one point of fixation to the next, blind to everything that happens during saccades. Or, you can slow your left and right glances down to close the gap between points of fixation and effectively decrease the time being blind to your surroundings.

Again, it goes back to what I wrote earlier (yes, I'm being repetitive): to see something accurately, you must look directly at it, and increase the fixation point interval by decreasing the saccade interval.

A trick I've taught myself is to mentally call out the color of the vehicles I'm watching. This takes only a microsecond but it's long enough to establish a point of fixation.

We Must Be Active Observers

The first step in making sure we don't become that accident victim is to make sure we are always actively observing our surroundings.

While this may sound obvious, many riders and drivers fail to do this. Let's go back to that four-way stop: We pull up to the stop sign, glance to our left, glance to our right — everything looks clear — and then move forward. We see the whole picture; a couple of cars stopped at the corner, buildings in the background, people on the sidewalk and the like, but what we need to see are the individual vehicles and pedestrians that might be a threat to us. We need to see past the surface-level big picture and observe more critically: do the drivers look like they're paying attention? Is that oncoming car going to blow the stop sign? Are the front wheels of the stopped cars moving forward ever so slightly? Is that pedestrian about to step off the curb? We can't see all these things with a quick glance; to see these things we must slow down our observation and actively look for them by directing our eyes to the specific areas in question and allowing enough time for fixation.

We must be active observers, well aware of the poor seeing habits of those around us. To protect ourselves, we must anticipate their gaps in sight before we fall victim to them.

Practice seeing defensively, and remember where we can make a big difference is with our own habits: Observe actively by looking directly at what you need to see; don't depend on peripheral vision and slow your glances down to reduce the duration of saccades and increase the points of fixation.

Further Repetition ('cause it's important!)

Remember, we see necessary detail within a very narrow range; specifically, two degrees on each side of center. Anything outside of that total of four degrees is noticed, but lacks detail. This becomes particularly important at intersections. If we only glance at traffic, rather than looking at it (establishing points of fixation) we can miss movement that might endanger us because, 1) we're not seeing it and, 2) it does not fall within those important four degrees.

In the example below, picture yourself sitting on the motorcycle. In sight line A, you are 75 feet from the car. At this distance your two degrees of detailed vision to each side of center (foveola vision) covers approximately 19 feet in width. Anything outside that width will not register as much detail. In sight line B you are seeing about 26 feet of width, and in sight line C about 16 feet.

In order to stay safe in this situation we need to *look* —not glance— at each intersection, and each element (car, pedestrian, bicycle, etc.) in it.

How much we actually see with our "foveola vision."

Sight Line Distance:
    A = 75 feet
    B = 100 feet
    C = 65 feet

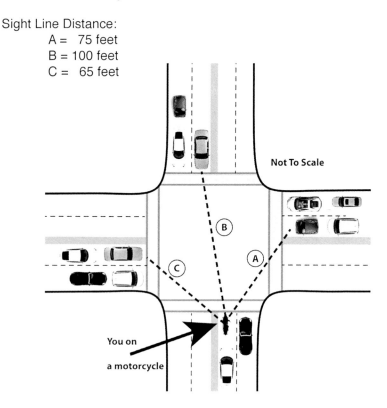

Night Riding

One of the first activities an aging motorcycle rider lets go of is night riding. As mentioned in Chapter 4, aging eyes that focus unevenly (anisometropia) and have yellowing of the lens or reduced pupil size all conspire to impair depth perception and reduce the amount of light that hits the retinas. All of this makes it increasingly difficult to discern color contrast and spot that shadowy deer that's lurking at the road's edge. It has been estimated that by age 60 the amount of light that reaches the photoreceptors in our retinas has been reduced by about two-thirds from that of when we were 20 years old. If we consider that the majority of the sensory information we need to be a competent rider is received by our eyes, it's obvious that any erosion of our eyesight could have a serious negative impact on our riding.

This erosion of vision is a normal — like it or not — function of aging, but it does not hit us all at the same age. For example, my night vision is still very good. It will get worse, but in this case I'm one of the more fortunate riders in my age group. Unfortunately, age can also bring about additional vision loss due to diseases such as glaucoma, cataracts, and retinopathy as a result of diabetes. The bottom line? Your night riding trips are numbered, but the age at which they'll end will differ from person to person.

That said, there is a way in which you might hold off this inevitability: Visit your eye doctor to find out the status of your vision, and if there are any medical steps that need be taken. Level with him. Tell him of any vision problems you might be experiencing, and explain that you are a motorcycle rider that occasionally rides at night. Assuming he gives you the OK to ride (grudgingly probably, as many medicos are not fond of their patients riding motorcycles) you can be confident that your night riding trips can be done safely.

See...

Motorcycle lighting technology has improved dramatically over the past several years, keeping pace with that of the automotive industry. While the technology has improved, its application to stock motorcycles is mostly limited to the headlight itself. Headlights are brighter, throw a pattern farther, and last longer than anything previously used, but they are still limited in their ability to light up the sides of the road, and are constrained by federal requirements restricting brightness. This is where auxiliary lights can provide significant benefit.

Four Different Lighting Technologies

There are four primary light technologies in play: incandescent, halogen, HID (high-intensity discharge), and LED (light-emitting diode). Many motorcycles are still equipped with incandescent lights, but this is a dead-end technology with roots reaching back to 1879 and Thomas Edison's first lightbulb. Incandescent light is produced when an electrical current is run through a tungsten filament causing the filament to glow. This method of lighting has had an admirable lifespan, but really can't compete with the other three technologies when it comes to efficiency and illumination.

Halogen lights are also incandescent lights, but their significantly smaller bulb contains halogen gas that allows for a much higher filament temperature and thus a much brighter light. Addition-ally, the life of

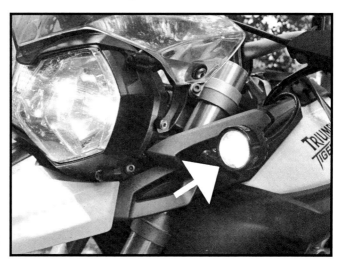

I run a set of Clearwater "Darla" LED lights on my Triumph. They pack 2000 lumens (that's a bunch) in a 2-inch package; very small but mighty. I highly recommend these lights.

a halogen bulb is usually at least twice that of a standard incandescent bulb. The downside to halogen lights is that they run very hot. This requires relatively heavy enclosures that act as a heat sink. They are also much more expensive than standard incandescent lights.

Rather than using a heated filament, HID lights (also called xenon lights) achieve their brightness via an electrical arc between two elec-trodes. This process can produce light that is up to three times brighter than the already very bright halogen lights, and is characterized by a bluish tint. These are probably the most annoying lights of any if you see them coming towards you, as their brightness and significant glare is very distracting. HID lights are very efficient, and last longer than halogen, but are also quite expensive.

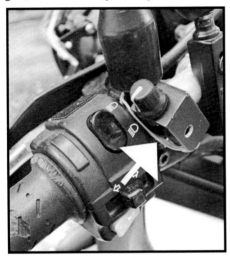

I control the intensity of the Clearwater lights via a rheostat mounted near my left grip.

The most recent lighting technology employs LEDs. The light from an LED comes from the production of photons (a basic light unit) as a result of the flow of electrons across a semi-conductor material. Lost? The science doesn't matter; all you need to know is that this method works very well, producing a bright light that falls between that of halogen and HID lights. Additionally, LEDs consume very little power, run cooler, and can be packed into very small containers. The big downside is that they are very expensive.

Auxiliary motorcycle lighting is available in incandescent, halogen, HID, and LED. Personally, my choice is LED, as incandescent lights do not provide the lighting I need, halogens generally run too hot, and HID lights really annoy those coming at you on the highway. It is very easy to find dissenting opinions on this, so if you're thinking of adding auxiliary lights, do your research and talk with riders who use the different types of lights.

A Note on Incandescent Lights

While my primary use for added lighting is to make my trips at night, or in failing light, all that much safer, there is a secondary reason that is almost as important: added lights tend to "paint" a larger picture of me during the day. ("Paint" is a techie term referring to the image size on a radar screen. For example, a Boeing 747 airplane "paints" a much larger image than does, say, a Cessna prop job.) I keep my auxiliary lights on during the day because they "paint" a larger picture of me to oncoming traffic, or the idiot who might make that left turn in front of me. If you ride only during the day, a good set of incandescent lights will work for this purpose, and save you a whole lot of money.

...And Be Seen

The picture I want to "paint" also applies from behind: I want to be seen by those drivers who are increasingly distracted by their stupidity (texting, calling, buttering their bagel…). Auxiliary lighting is also available for the rear, and I particularly recommend any that work in conjunction with the brake light (as opposed to just being running lights). There are two primary ways to add auxiliary rear lights. The first is to modify your turn signals to work with your brake light. They will still function as turn signals, but those following you will see three lights flash (instead of one) when you hit the rear brake. The second method is to add aftermarket lights that work as both running lights and brake lights.

There is another route to make yourself more visible at night, and it's relatively inexpensive: reflective tape. SOLAS is an acronym referring to "Safety Of Life At Sea." It is a set of requirements, determined by members of the International Maritime Organization, specifying minimum standards for construction, equipment, and operation of ships. As a part of their outlined standards they require reflective tape be used on life rafts, immersion suits, railings, life jackets… anything that needs to be seen.

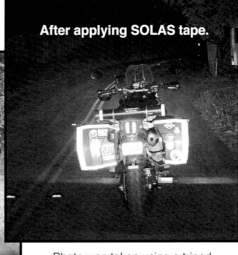

After applying SOLAS tape.

The rear of my Triumph with no SOLAS tape applied.

Photo was taken using a tripod, no flash. The SOLAS tape has lit up due to the focusing laser from the camera and the taillight.

Don't Go for Cheap Imitations

There are few environments as harsh as life at sea. Water, corrosive salts, and baking sun are the major elements that attack anything and everything on and in the water. Because of this, the standard for marine-grade reflective tape far surpasses any condition that it might face on land. The result of these standards is SOLAS-grade tape, also known as retroreflective tape. This is a very rugged, highly reflective tape that, when hit by headlights, shines as if it were a bank of bright lights. When applied to the rear of your motorcycle, approaching traffic will see you. As shown in the photos I have outlined my saddlebags with SOLAS tape. Very similar to SOLAS-grade tape is Prismatic Tape; a tape made from the same material used on reflective stop signs. Neither one of these products are cheap, but both are well worth the cost in keeping the rear end of your motorcycle — not to mention your own — safe from damage. Despite the cost, pay it: this is not a place to save money. While the cheap tape might provide similar reflectivity, it will not survive the rigors of sun and rain. One last thing on these tapes: Be sure and locate them where you want them to be. There are no do-overs as the tape is very difficult to remove.

Mirrors

Being able to see behind you can often be as important as seeing what's ahead. This is particularly true in stop-and-go traffic. There are few riding experiences more painful than having a following car stop about two feet into the rear of your motorcycle. Just as important, is being able to see what lurks to each side when you want to make a lane change. At this time, the most reasonable and reliable defense we have against becoming a hood ornament is our rearview mirrors. In the case of a lane change, add in a twist of the head.

It has been a long-standing tradition among motorcycle manufacturers to equip their products with pathetically ineffective mirrors that can best be used for stunning views of our elbows. These mirrors are not designed for function, just style. No designer wants to disrupt their styling effort by tacking on a pair of Mickey Mouse ears, so they often design barely adequate appendages that meet the letter of the law but little else. Fortunately, this trend is changing, particularly with touring and adventure motorcycles. There are three things you can do to help improve rearward vision. If you're happy with the size of your mirrors, but find your body blocking part of the view, you can extend the mirror stalks. These extensions are available for most all motorcycles and take the form of an inexpensive insert which screws in between the mirror mount and the existing stalk. If you want to improve the range of the mirror's movement, articulated mounts are also available.

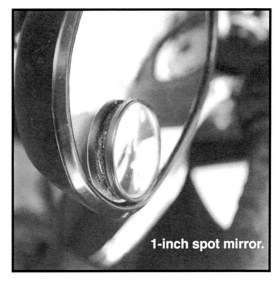

1-inch spot mirror.

The next step you can take is to replace your too-small mirrors with oversized units. Again, these are available for most models of motorcycles. If you are happy with the size of your mirrors and they extend out sufficiently, there is another way to increase your

The next step you can take is to replace your too-small mirrors with oversized units. Again, these are available for most models of motorcycles. If you are happy with the size of your mirrors and they extend out sufficiently, there is another way to increase your field of view: attach a "spot" mirror to either or both of your mirrors. These are small convex mirrors that bulge

It has been a long-standing tradition among motorcycle manufacturers to equip their products with pathetically ineffective mirrors.

outwards to give you a wider view of what's behind or beside you. These mirrors can be easily attached to your stock mirrors via double-sided tape. They are available in various sizes and shapes, but I've found that a 1-inch round works well. Take note: Because of their convex shape, these mirrors make vehicles look farther away than they really are.

The next technological step on the horizon for rearward viewing is small high-resolution cameras that feed a remote screen attached to your dash or handlebar. There are a few units currently available, but I've not been impressed with the quality (which is why I've yet to try one). Additionally, there is at least one helmet manufacturer that will shortly release a camera-equipped helmet with a heads-up display. As I write this, it is undergoing beta testing on the heads of carefully selected riders.

Rain Riding

There's a somewhat regular conversation that takes place in the Kittrelle household. It goes something like this…

You taking the bike?

Yeah.

But it's raining!

Hey, it's what I do.

I wouldn't say that I *like* riding in the rain, but it usually doesn't bother me all that much, and I seldom avoid it because I look at wet riding as part of keeping my skills sharp.

There are two ways to approach wet weather riding: with fear or respect. If you fear it, don't do it, unless you must — and then figure out a way to not do it. Yes, I know all about facing down one's fears, but if riding a motorcycle is a somewhat casual, fair-weather activity for you there is no real reason to put yourself at increased risk. This is a classic example of risk assessment: do your needs to ride in the rain outweigh the involved risks? If the answer is no, then simply don't do it. If yes, then you need to work on changing your fear into respect.

Dressing for Your Riding Event

The first step to prepare for rain riding begins before you climb in the saddle, and involves dressing properly. A distracted rider is an unsafe rider, and a trickle of cold water running down our spine can be a big distraction — not to mention how distracting a wet crotch, soggy gloves and a fogged-up face shield can be. There is a wealth of excellent wet-weather riding gear on the market, but it all suffers from the same fault: it wasn't designed for you… or me. Out of necessity, clothing manufacturers design to fit the average rider, a mythical person that I have never come across. We humans come in a wide variety of sizes and shapes, which don't always fit that "average" pattern. The jacket is your key piece of gear and is the most difficult

There are two ways to approach wet weather riding: with fear or respect.

to fit properly. Generally, this is not a problem in fair-weather riding as a snug collar or proper-length sleeves don't always matter that much. The rain changes this. If your collar is too loose, water will find its way in. If you're collar is too tight, you won't close it, and water will find a way in. If your sleeves aren't the proper length they can make a good wrist seal difficult and water will find a way in. Regardless of the item of clothing, you will find fit glitches that can ruin your wet riding day.

The way to solve these fit problems is to take along your riding gear when you try on new jackets at the dealer. This means your helmet, gloves, neck warmer, heated liner — anything that you will be using under the jacket you want to buy. Some of the problems I have found with otherwise excellent jackets include neck closures that don't close when I'm wearing a neck warmer because the Velcro tab is just too short, and cuffs that

There is a wealth of excellent wet weather riding gear on the market, but it all suffers from the same fault: it wasn't designed for you… or me.

won't properly close over my heated liner. In one case, I couldn't close my left cuff because it wouldn't fit over my watch. In fact, the match-up of gloves and jacket cuffs can be a big problem because the gauntlet part of gloves often refuses to fit over jacket cuffs. Pants can also be a bit of a problem, with one of my biggest complaints being with those overpants that require you to remove your boots before taking the overpants off; a rider did not design pants like those.

Helmets can also be problematic in rain weather. Two major issues you might encounter are rainwater running down the inside of your face shield (due to a bad fit at the brow level) and fogging of the shield. Once you've purchased the helmet there's little you can do about this fit problem, so be sure and eyeball it closely before you buy it, looking for any gaps between the top of the shield and the sealing grommet. (Note: some of the better helmets have an adjustment that will close that gap.) If you are stuck with this situation, a temporary fix is to stuff a thin section of paper towel in the gap between the shield and the helmet. Eliminating fogging can be tricky. There are several different products on the market that claim to eliminate this problem, but my experience is that sometimes they work, and sometimes they don't. Which is why I am not recommending any. To get around this, I wear clear glasses that allow me to slightly crack the shield to let in a fog-dispersing breeze.

By wearing your gear while trying on possible new jackets and pants you can be assured that once the rain starts you'll remain focused and dry.

Dealing With the Fear of Rain

Like most fears, that of rain riding is overstated in your mind with the reality of it being far less scary. If you've chosen to face this fear, rather than avoiding rain riding, you'll need, first, to change your approach to it. That is, look at it as another challenge and an excellent way to add to your bank of motorcycle skills.

Dealing with the fear —or call it anxiety if it makes you feel better— of actually riding in the rain starts with a deep breath. One of our body's quirks is that when we are anxious or fearful, we have a tendency to tense up and take only shallow breaths. This classic fight, flight, or freeze response is a normal response to anxiety. The beneficial aspect of this response is that it increases the flow of adrenaline, clarifies our thinking, and forces us to focus on the job at hand. However, in order to reap its benefits, we need to get this response under control; a tensed-up body, deprived of oxygen, can lead to all manner of problems on a motorcycle including over-reaction to input. Getting this anxiety under control is fairly simple. As you sit in the saddle, getting ready to thumb the starter, take a couple of deep breaths. Focus on letting each breath out completely. You will feel more relaxed as this brief exercise helps to relieve the tension in your body and focus your mind.

> **Primary Rain Rules**
>
> 1. Slow Down
> 2. Increase your following distance

The primary rules when heading out onto a wet highway are: 1) slow down and, 2) increase your following distance. There is a third rule that can come in handy: do everything in one gear higher. How you approach this third rule will depend upon how your motorcycle is geared, but the idea behind this is that by clicking up one gear you remove some of the abruptness of the lower gear, which can help to maintain traction.

Because of reduced traction in the wet, failure to follow rules number one and two are a great set-up towards you and your motorcycle face planting into the rear of the car you're following. According to the Motorcycle Safety Foundation, stopping distances for motorcycles and cars, in the dry, on a straight clean road, are "nearly" equal. Throw rain on the road, however, and the stopping distance advantage swings clearly to the car. Despite the much heavier car weight, the relatively small tire contact "footprint" of motorcycle tires cannot compete with the much larger footprint of even the smallest car tires. Because of this, I generally increase my rain-riding following distance by double or triple my normal dry-conditions distance. In some cases it can be significantly more, such as when the spray from the vehicle ahead obscures my vision. While doing this will keep you safe(r) it can also create yet another problem — tailgating by the car behind you. Many car drivers have a totally unreal-

A wet highway brings out all sorts of things to be avoided, or at least to be dealt with differently than when dry.

istic view of motorcycles and what they can do, particularly regarding stopping distances. This often means that the twit behind you can't understand why you've backed off, so they respond by riding your tail. Do not close up your following distance to make them happy. If possible, let them pass. If that can't happen, I've found that a serious "Back off!" wave usually brings them to their senses. Another often-effective ploy is to turn on your emergency flashers for a brief period. If all else fails, pull to the side of the road and let them go. To do otherwise is to guarantee that your two wheels are going to seriously lose against even the smallest of four wheels.

The smooth operation of a motorcycle pays dividends regardless of the weather, but in reduced traction situations smoothness becomes even more important. Abrupt lane changes, slamming the throttle open or closed, and grabbing a handful of brake can easily break traction, and contribute to an expensive ambulance ride. Something else to understand about wet riding is that once you've lost traction it becomes very difficult, if not impossible, to get it back. That fun slide on dry pavement becomes a not-so-fun crash in the wet.

If You Can't Avoid the Rain, Avoid These

A wet highway brings out all sorts of things to be avoided, or at least to be dealt with differently than when dry. The first thing to avoid, if possible, is riding at all after a long dry spell. Give the rain a chance to wash away the accumulated dirt, oil, and rubber from the road before you set a wheel on it. Once out there, be very aware of anything painted or applied to the road surface as the available traction can be close to zero. This would include crosswalks, directional arrows, centerlines and diamond-shaped commuter lane (HOV) markers. Originally, all these various marking were done with paint, but over the years advancing technology has replaced most painted markings with a plastic or epoxy mixture. These are cheaper and more reflective, but if crossed at a lean they will put a motorcycle on the ground faster than you can say, "What the...?"

Another 20 Million Things to Avoid

There are a few other noteworthy items on which to ride very carefully, including manhole covers, railroad tracks, any metal, reflective markers and raised highway bumps known as "Bott's Dots." Manhole covers and railroad tracks are also particularly evil (wet or dry); always be sure to cross them straight up in the saddle. Bott's Dots were invented by Dr. Elbert D. Botts of California's Department of Transportation (Cal-Trans) back in 1953. The idea is that when a vehicle drifts over them, it gets the driver's attention. Hit a set of them while leaned over in a turn,

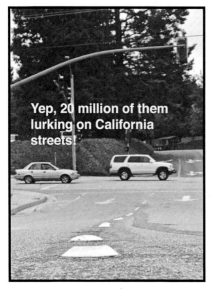

Yep, 20 million of them lurking on California streets!

and they'll get a rider's attention, post haste! I'd say avoid them completely, but according to CalTrans more than 20 million of them are in place just in California alone.

One of the most obvious dangers of riding in the rain is standing water. This is a particular problem when rain first begins because drains are often blocked with debris. A good way to manage this hazard is by keeping your speed down, as the faster you hit a puddle, the more likely you are to hydroplane. As the term implies, to hydroplane means your front wheel can lose contact with the road causing it to barely skim, or plane, across the water (hydro), which leads to an all-out loss of steering ability. If you hydroplane in a turn, you're down. Period. No questions asked. If you hit a large puddle on the straight, the way out of that problem is to gently slow down, stay off the front brake, and steer straight ahead. Above all, don't take your feet off the pegs (in hope of adding stability) as this does nothing more than raise the center of gravity, making it all the more likely you'll incur a splashdown.

and this... Rain Hack

If you live in the Pacific Northwest or similarly, uh, damp places, you probably always pack along rain gear. Riders in drier climes can generally consider the time of year when deciding whether to carry rain gear, but it can be a gamble. If you do get caught without your waterproof gear there is a simple, surprisingly effective hack: plastic garbage bags.

Use a large size for your body. Cut a neck opening at the bottom of the bag just large enough to get your head through, and a similar opening at each corner for your arms. Wear the body bag under your jacket. If you wear it over your jacket, the wind will shred it, and it provides far less warmth. Slip a small bag over each sock then put on your boots. Make sure to run the bags as far up your legs as they will go. If you roll it down from your boot tops, it will channel water into your boots.

Because these plastic bags do not breathe, you'll find they can keep you quite warm (and sweaty) which makes them handy not only in wet weather, but also on cold days.

Napping

Did you know that we old folks have a "Day?" Yep, it is October 1 of each year, "The International Day of Older Persons." It was first observed in 1991 as a day to appreciate just what us old codgers have contributed to the world. I don't recall anyone ever toasting me, or laying a gift on me in past Octobers, so I wouldn't get too excited about this. There is, however, what you might call a related day of celebration worth mentioning. It is the day after the spring return of Daylight Savings Time: National Napping Day. Taking a nap often gets a bad rap because, well, only babies and old people need naps, right? Wrong. Research actually shows that everyone can benefit from a nap even when it's not National Napping Day.

The National Sleep Foundation (NSF) identifies three types of naps:

1) **Planned napping** (preparatory napping) involves taking a nap before you actually get sleepy. You may use this technique when you know that you will be up later than your normal bedtime or as a mechanism to ward off getting tired earlier.

2) **Emergency napping** occurs when you are suddenly very tired and cannot continue with the activity you were originally engaged in. This type of nap can be used to combat drowsy riding or fatigue while using heavy and dangerous machinery.

3) **Habitual napping** is practiced when a person takes a nap at the same time each day. Young children may fall asleep at about the same time each afternoon or an adult might take a short nap after lunch each day.

More importantly, the NSF highlights several benefits derived from napping:

• Naps can restore alertness, enhance performance, and reduce mistakes and accidents. A study at NASA on sleepy military pilots and astronauts found that a 40-minute nap improved performance by 34 percent and alertness by 100 percent.

• Naps can increase alertness in the period directly following the nap and may extend alertness a few hours later in the day.

• Scheduled napping has also been prescribed for those who are affected by narcolepsy.

• Napping has psychological benefits. A nap can be a pleasant luxury, a mini-vacation. It can provide an easy way to get some relaxation and rejuvenation.

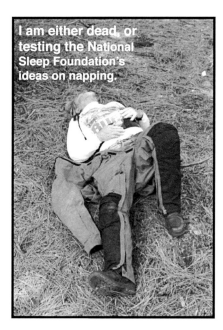

I am either dead, or testing the National Sleep Foundation's ideas on napping.

There are, however, some caveats related to napping. Expert opinion has settled on the fact that short naps — 30 minutes in length at most — carry the most benefit. If you zonk out longer than this, you risk impacting that important good night's sleep that you need. The longer the nap, the longer it takes to wake up from it. You know that groggy, zombie-like feeling? That's called sleep inertia, and it can take a while to wear off.

Don't fight the feeling. If you're holding sleep at arm's length, give into it. This is particularly true if you're on a motorcycle trip. There have been several occasions that I have stretched out on a rest stop bench, and grabbed a 10-minute nap. Napping is good for your mind and your body, and riding zoned-out or sleep deprived isn't good for anyone.

and this... Sleep

There are four primary stages of sleep. The first three are defined as Non-REM sleep with REM standing for "rapid eye movement." The REM state of sleep is the deepest sleep level and is often characterized by intense dreams. By the way, the "rapid eye movement" is well documented, but the reasons for it remain unclear.

Non-REM Sleep

Stage 1: The first stage of sleep. Easy to wake from with people often not realizing they were asleep.

Stage 2: Light sleep; easily awakened, awareness fades.

Stage 3: Deep sleep begins; difficult to wake up.

REM Sleep

Accounts for about 25% of adult sleep time; cycles in and out throughout the night in periods up to about 90 minutes. Deep sleep, Intense dreaming.

in other words

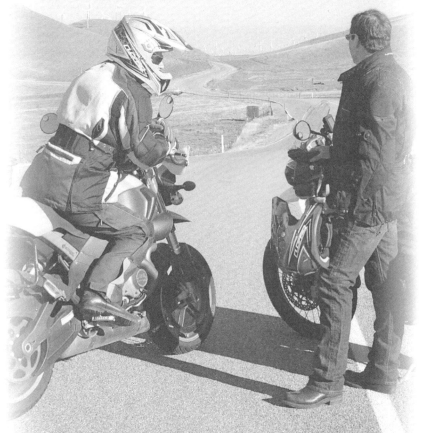

Rick Diaz

Rick Diaz, 56

I never stopped to think what it would be like to be an older rider...

Little did I know back when I was 13 and having my first-ever ride on that Honda Mini-Trail 50 that it would begin a relationship with motorcycles that would last my entire life. Since the age of 17 I have never not owned a motorcycle of some form. Now, at 56, I can look back on a two-wheeled history that included many dirt bikes, ATVs, and all manner of street motorcycles from sportbikes to my current touring bike. While I was collecting memories and embellishing tales of derring-do, I never stopped to think what it would be like to be an older rider and the ramifications age would have on my ability to ride. I'm starting to think of those things, now, like it or not.

Having not been just a rider, but also a motocross racer, motorcycle shop owner and traveling motojournalist, I have had more than my fair share of adventures —and misadventures— on two wheels. I have the hardware and scars to show for the latter, as well. These days, it doesn't take much to remind me how I got each and every one of them. A damp day and my knees are tied in knots. A sudden drop in temperature and my back sounds like an old Craftsman ratchet

Even with all my aches and pains, that 13-year-old boy on a mini bike inside me just wants to keep riding for as long as the road (and my body) will let me.

wrench. These days, riding is more like an exercise in trying to keep my body parts from their cacophonous clattering. A symphony in B minor, so to speak (the B standing for Bone). The dirt bike is gone as I no longer wish to put another orthopedist's child through college. The last sport-bike, a Buell I lovingly customized myself is also gone, at the insistence of my back, arms and shoulders that could no longer find an amicable resolution to its riding posture. All that remains is my trusty Harley touring bike with its wide saddle and neutral seating position. A reward for having made it to the ranks of AARP membership.

I no longer ride long distance as I once could, and since moving from California to Florida I ride even less due to the unbearable heat of

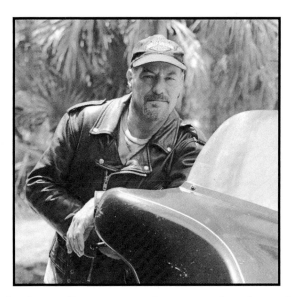

summer or the threat of spontaneous downpours that plague this state much of the year. But still, I ride. Riding motorcycles has been the only constant in my adult life and I love it like nothing else. Through marriages and divorces, good times and bad, motorcycling has always been there for me. I still get a thrill when I throw my leg over a bike and hear that engine roar. As cliché as it sounds, the feeling of the open road …the wind in my face …the freedom of being on two wheels, is still something my body, mind and soul crave. Deeply. Even with all my aches and pains, that 13-year-old boy on a mini bike inside me just wants to keep riding for as long as the road (and my body) will let me.

Tools 101

DRILL PRESS: A tall upright machine useful for suddenly snatching flat metal bar stock out of your hands so that it smacks you in the chest and flings your beer across the room, denting the freshly painted project which you had carefully set in the corner where nothing could get to it.

WIRE WHEEL: Cleans paint off bolts and then throws them somewhere under the workbench with the speed of light. Also removes fingerprints and hard-earned calluses from fingers.

PLIERS: Used to round off bolt heads. Sometimes used in the creation of blood blisters.

HACKSAW: One of a family of cutting tools built on the Ouija board principle... It transforms human energy into a crooked, unpredictable motion, and the more you attempt to influence its course, the more dismal your future becomes.

VISE-GRIPS: Generally used after pliers to completely round off bolt heads. If nothing else is available, they can also be used to transfer intense welding heat to the palm of your hand.

OXYACETYLENE TORCH: Used almost entirely for lighting various flammable objects in your shop on fire. Also handy for igniting the grease inside the wheel hub out of which you want to remove a bearing race.

PHILLIPS SCREWDRIVER: Normally used to stab the vacuum seals under lids or for opening old-style paper-and-tin oil cans and splashing oil on your shirt; but can also be used, as the name implies, to strip out Phillips screw heads.

STRAIGHT SCREWDRIVER: A tool for opening paint cans. Sometimes used to convert common slotted screws into non-removable screws and butchering your palms.

PRY BAR: A tool used to crumple the metal surrounding that clip or bracket you needed to remove in order to replace a 50 cent part.

HOSE CUTTER: A tool used to make hoses too short.

HAMMER: Originally employed as a weapon of war, the hammer nowadays is used as a kind of divining rod to locate the most expensive parts adjacent the object we are trying to hit.

UTILITY KNIFE: Used to open and slice through the contents of cardboard cartons delivered to your front door; works particularly well on contents such as seats, vinyl records, liquids in plastic bottles, collector magazines, refund checks, and rubber or plastic parts. Especially useful for slicing work clothes, but only while in use.

WHITWORTH SOCKETS: Once used for working on older British cars and motorcycles, they are now used mainly for impersonating that 9/16 or 1/2 inch socket you've been searching for the last 45 minutes.

PHONE: Tool for calling an ambulance.

Tried to find the author of this, but there are several different versions. So, to the anonymous You, Thanx! R.K.

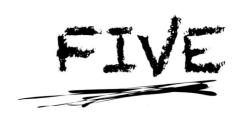

hardware...

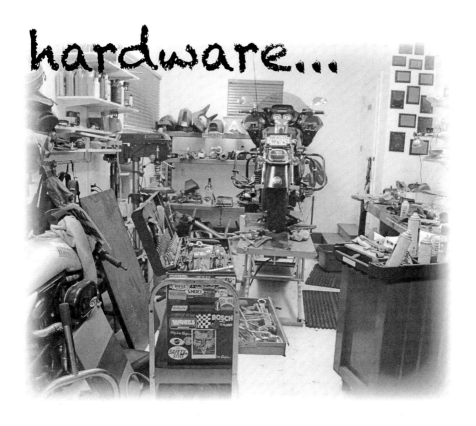

14.

Duct tape is like the Force. It has a light side,
a dark side, and it holds the universe together.

Anon.

Tools for Bike and Body

Yet another change that we older riders have experienced is a shift in the discussion of tools. In particular, which ones should we carry with us? In addition to my "Fix-It Kit" (see sidebar) I carry Vise-Grips, duct tape, a Leatherman "Surge" multi-tool, a cell phone, and a credit card. These items will largely — if not completely — cover just about everything I'd need in the event of a twenty-first century breakdown.

Today's motorcycles are highly dependable. And very complex. What this translates to is that they very seldom break down, but when they do… it's generally game over, call the tow truck. The days of burnishing ignition points and cleaning out carburetor float bowls by the side of the road are long gone. Does this mean that it's unnecessary to pack along tools? No, what it means is that the tools we now carry should reflect today's need, not tradition.

If your motorcycle stops running there are a few obvious things you can check right away. Do you have gas? With large gas tanks and good gas mileage, riders have been known to overlook the gas gauge. How about the battery? Battery life is significantly longer than it once was, and with the battery usually buried under various panels, we have a tendency to forget about it. Other than those two things, about all else you can do is a close visual of, primarily, electrical components like fuses, wiring, and spark plug leads. One indispensable tool you're never without can be helpful if there's an electrical problem: your nose. Shorted wires can happen, and often emit a noticeable burn smell. This is particularly true if you've added any electrical farkles such as auxiliary lights or a power outlet. If the wiring to these items is unfused (Bad you!) and a short occurs, it will blow the fuse attached to the line into which you spliced; a fuse that might be critical to the operation of the motorcycle.

Fixing Our Mistakes

The tools that you do carry should be focused on the mistakes you might make, not the unlikely failures of the manufacturer. And mistakes requiring tools usually means you've managed to lay the bike down... and maybe not too gently. Assuming you're unhurt, the tools you'll need are those that can straighten bent levers, remove shattered cladding, and secure or remove damaged nonessentials, such as turn signals, mirrors and saddlebags.

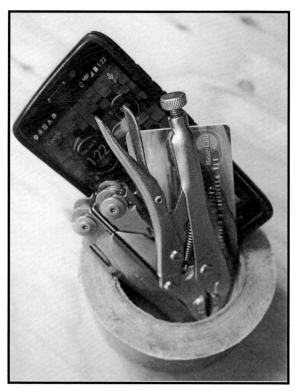

If I were restricted to carrying only three items, they would be Vise-Grips, a roll of Gorilla tape (extra strong duct tape), and a Leatherman Surge multi-tool. I've named brands because these specific products have stood

Today's basic tool kit.

the test of various trials with me. The Vise-Grips can be used to lock on to sheared hand or foot lever stubs, and duct tape needs no explanation. I like the Leatherman Surge because it has large pliers and a good assortment of tools and blades.

For anything that can't be fixed with Vise-Grips, duct tape, Leatherman, or a fix-it kit, I'll break open the cellphone/credit card combo.

The Basic Fix-It Kit Checklist

___   Wiring diagram

___   6 feet 16 ga. galvanized steel wire
> (Strong; can replace a missing through-bolt)

___   6 feet 14 ga. stranded electrical wire

___   Small roll heavy-duty duct tape

___   Roll electrical tape

___   Assorted zip ties

___   Fuse set

___   Large Vise-Grips

___   Torx wrenches (Specific to your motorcycle; not the whole set!)

___   Hex wrenches (ditto)

___   Blade and Phillips screwdrivers

___   Sidecutters

___   8-inch adjustable wrench

___   Combination wrenches
> (The wrenches you carry will fall into two categories:
> Those necessary to remove front and rear wheels and
> those necessary to remove and replace broken or
> failed items.)

___ Multi-tool

___ LED flashlight

___ Multi-meter (Use to test for open/shorted wires, fuses, etc.)

___ Shop rag

___ Plug kit for tubeless tires with 6 to 8 CO2 cartridges
> or a 12v air pump
>> (Note: The quantity of CO2 cartridges found in many plug
>> kits are insufficient to pump up a tire.)

or…

___ Tube-type tire tools:
> Bead-breaking tools
>
> Tire irons
>
> Patch kit
>
> 12v air pump

and this... Duct Tape

It's 1973 and Chris and I are riding the annual off-road Cow Bell enduro in Northern California, with about 10 miles left to the finish. It's been raining all day and the trails are little more than mud troughs. As we approach yet another brush-covered muddy hill climb we can see that the thick goo is moving like a slow-motion landslide. It isn't a long climb, but it is obvious that momentum is needed to overcome the mud flow.

We hit the base of the hill at speed, keeping the bikes moving upward at a steady pace. As we near the top, my brake level snags on something. This stops my bike instantly, slams my chest into the handlebars, and tosses me on my back into the mud with my head pointing downhill. I hurt, and the mud is creeping over me. With Chris's help I am able to sit up, but anything more than shallow breaths creates a stabbing pain in my chest. It's obvious that a couple of ribs have been broken. This is a bit of a problem because cellphones hadn't been invented yet, and we are 20 miles from help.

Slowly, I am able to get to my feet, and I'm OK as long as I don't breathe deeply or move quickly. Riding the bike? Problematic, but I don't have a lot of choices. I don't recall which one of us came up with the idea, but as always we're both carrying a roll of that indispensable item, duct tape. I need to keep my chest as immovable as possible, so Chris wraps my torso in the tape. There is no way I can remove my jacket, so he wraps the tape around me as an outer layer.

Suitably mummified, I felt a bit better. Chris kickstarts my motorcycle, and I gingerly climb aboard. Snicking it into gear, I ease out the clutch and begin the slow, painful ride to the finish.

Without the duct tape I would have not been able to do that.

What did I learn? Cellphones are good. Duct tape is essential. I always carry both.

Selecting and Maintaining Batteries

Let's revisit batteries. Years ago batteries were a continual source of problems with motorcycles because battery life was not particularly good. The two primary reasons for this were marginal battery quality and motorcycle vibration that caused batteries to — more or less — shake and crack themselves to death.

Today, both batteries and motorcycles are so well made that we tend to forget about them. Generally, a two-year life for a well-maintained conventional battery is no problem. Sealed batteries (more on these below) should see three to four years of life. Yuasa, the largest distributor of motorcycle batteries in the U.S., says that six to eight years of life for a well-maintained sealed battery is possible.

Maintenance for non-sealed batteries is a cinch if you ride regularly; all you really need do is keep the terminals clean and secure, and periodically checked the fluid level. It is also important to coat the terminals — particularly the mating surfaces — with an anti-corrosive compound that's easily found at auto parts stores. Corrosion on the mating surfaces raises the electrical resistance and reduces voltage flow. Too much corrosion on loose terminals can cause the voltage from your battery to fall below the required minimum level. Be careful when cleaning the corrosion, as its chemical makeup is lead sulfate, a toxic chemical. Also know that the terminals on your battery are made from lead, and that metal, because of its softness, has a tendency to "flow" and deform to the point where the connections becomes loose; check your terminal health regularly.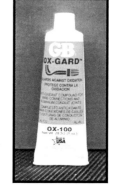

If you only ride once a month or so (perish the thought!) or weather keeps your motorcycle in storage for extended periods, the investment in a battery trickle charger is less expensive than buying a new battery. Charging a battery is not necessarily as simple as it might seem. Read on, and I'll highlight the issues with charging. First, a bit of battery basics.

Comparing Different Types of Batteries

Despite the very rapid advance of battery technology in recent years (Thank you Zero, Brammo, Tesla...) the lead-acid type, invented by Gaston Plante back in 1859, still remains the most widely used.

The packaging and internals have changed over the years, but voltage generation still depends upon the flow of electrons through an electrolyte (battery acid) between positive and negative lead plates. Hence, the name lead-acid battery, or, as they're occasionally called, "wet cell" batteries.

VRLA: Gel or AGM

For riders, one of the biggest improvements with these batteries was introduction of the VRLA (valve-regulated lead-acid) motorcycle-specific battery by Yuasa in the mid-1980's. This technology replaced the removable filler screws on traditional batteries with a single pressure relief valve. It also eliminated the messy — and often damaging— process of refilling battery cells. These batteries are a boon to customizers as they can be oriented in any position except upside down. VRLA batteries are available in two different versions: Gel and AGM (absorbed glass mat). These two types of VRLA batteries are often mistaken for each other so pay attention, as there are important differences.

Gel VRLA batteries replace the battery-acid electrolyte with a thick jellylike substance, while AGM VRLA batteries use a spongelike glass mat to hold a relatively small amount of electrolyte. AMG batteries are the most common amongst motorcycle batteries. For our purposes we don't need to jump into the chemistry behind how these batteries work, but it is important that you understand how these two batteries differ from one another. For the casual, fair-weather rider, either a Gel or AGM battery should work just fine. If you fall outside the casual/fair-weather rider parameters, or if you live in a cold climate and ride throughout the year, an AGM battery is the better option as it is not as prone to lose power in low temperatures as are the Gel types. Even more important, an AGM battery is preferred if you're loaded up with watt-sucking accessories such as a GPS, auxiliary lighting, smart phone, or heated clothing.

Lithium-ion Batteries

The newest, to date, battery technology is lithium-ion (Li-ion). First introduced for commercial products in 1991, Li-ion batteries are now used in most consumer electronics such as phones and computers and are available in numerous configurations, including those for motorcycles. Li-ion batteries are actually a class of batteries as there are at least a half a dozen types, with the difference between each battery being internal chemistry. Li-ion batteries designated for motorcycle use fall into the Lithium Iron Phosphate (LIFePO4) class. There are several advantages to Li-ion batteries over lead-acid. One that is instantly notice-able before you install it is weight. The internal electrode plates are made from lithium and iron phosphate-coated carbon rather than the tradition lead. Lithium is the lightest of all pure metals (some alloys are lighter) and carbon weighs next to nothing, as we all know from those pricey carbon-fiber pieces that dot our motorcycles. I recently installed a Shorai LFX Li-ion battery in my Triumph Tiger. The OE Yuasa battery weighed 11 pounds, 8 ounces; the replace-ment Shorai came in at 3 pounds, 3 ounces. That is a significant weight savings that — in my case — makes a pretty significant difference as the bat-tery in my Triumph sits above the bike's center of gravity.

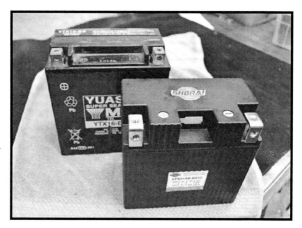

The Lithium-ion battery, at front, weighs more than 8 pounds *less* than the similarly-sized lead-acid battery at the rear.

While a weight savings is nice to have, the real benefit to Li-ion batteries is their energy density, or, in other words, just how much energy their given system can contain. This is commonly measured in watt-hours, with one watt-hour of power being expended for one hour of time. For example, a standard lead-acid bat-tery can store approximately 25 watt-hours per kilogram (2.2 pounds) of battery weight: a typical Li-ion battery can store 150 watt-hours per kilogram.

The downside to Li-ion technology, relative to lead-acid batteries, is that you have to pay a bit more attention to them. Specifically, you must not run them down to nothing or they won't recharge and you must not overcharge a Li-ion battery or you'll destroy it. They do, however, hold a charge for a very long time. Typically, sitting idle (no load on it) a lead-acid battery will lose 4 percent to 6 percent of its power monthly, whereas a Li-ion battery will lose only 2 percent to 3 percent.

Surf the net and you'll see some complaints about Li-ion Shorai failure in cold weather, but this probably has more to do with folks not keeping the battery on a trickle charger when the motorcycle sits unused for long periods.

Battery Charging Tips

Motorcycle batteries can be very expensive, ranging in price from under $100 for small motorcycles to well over $300 for some Li-ion batteries. If maintained properly a quality battery can be expected to last several years. If a battery doesn't last that long, the cause can often be traced back to us — the riders.

The single biggest factor in battery death is sulfation. This is the build up of a chemical on the internal electrode plates that serves to block the flow of electrons between the plates. A major cause of this is not keeping a trickle charger (aka float charger) on the battery while your motorcycle sits idle for long periods of time. Generally speaking, if you don't ride for more than two weeks at a time, its best to keep that box of volts on a charger. As I mentioned above, your common lead-acid battery loses between 4 percent and 6 percent of its power per month when it's sitting doing nothing. Typically, a fully charged battery should show a minimum of 12.6 volts, so that loss percentage calculates to between 0.5 volts and 0.75 volts. Add in the power draw from items that require

The safest way around battery charging problems is to use a smart charger.

power even when the ignition is off, such as an alarm system and radio (gotta keep the internal clock ticking along), and that power loss percentage creeps up.

Another battery killer is overcharging. This usually results from the use of an incorrect charger that boils the electrolyte mass away. Potentially (but rare) this can be fatal to living things, not just your battery, as the boiling electrolyte creates hydrogen, which is flammable when mixed with oxygen.

The safest way around battery charging problems is to use a "smart charger." They're called "smart" because, rather than just charging your battery, they continually monitor the state of the charge. This assures that the battery is properly charged, given its size in amps, and prevents overcharging. Additionally, a "smart charger" can function as a trickle charger to maintain the battery of a stored motorcycle. If you are using a

Gel battery, you will require a charger designed for these types of batteries as the recharge voltage required is much lower than that of lead-acid and AGM batteries. If you use a charger other than a Gel charger — even if you use the Gel setting on your smart charger — you risk overcharging the battery and severely shortening its life. Lithium-ion batteries also require a special charger as they cannot accept any degree of overcharge without suffering damage. Some smart chargers are capable of charging Li-ion batteries, but before you stick your Li-ion battery on there, make sure you read all the instructions that come with the charger.

While smart chargers are typically more expensive than standard battery chargers — and Li-ion chargers even more expensive — they are overall cheaper than having to replace a damaged battery.

Battery Load Capacity

There is yet another battery issue that you need be concerned with, and it should be of particular concern with touring motorcycles: load capacity. While it's not necessary here to launch a full explanation of motorcycle electrical systems, it is important that you understand the capacity of your motorcycle's electrical system to power add-on accessories.

The purpose of a motorcycle alternator is to maintain a proper voltage level in the battery, and to power anything and everything that runs on electricity. This "anything and everything" can be defined as either operating load or accessory load. Operating load is what your motorcycle requires to, well, operate. This includes the ignition, fuel injection, headlight, tail and brake lights, microprocessors, and instrument lighting.

Accessory load is what you draw from the battery to operate the accessories that you've added to the system. If you're a Farkle Fanatic this list can get lengthy, but the most popular items include auxiliary lighting, GPS system, MP3 player, cell phone charger, radar detector, and heated clothing (liner, pants, gloves, socks, etc.).

The power supplied to each item, in each category, depends upon what each item needs. This need is usually expressed in watts. For example, it's not unusual for a heated jacket liner to require 100 watts of power. This is referred to as its power "draw," as it draws that much from the electrical system. Every motorcycle alternator has a maximum power output, expressed in watts or amps-hours (Ah). If you attempt to draw more power than the alternator can supply, not only will your lights, ignition, and electrical accessories not function properly, but you will also suck the life out of your battery. To forestall this, you need to do a bit of simple electrical load calculation.

Step one is to determine the peak output of your alternator. This information can usually be found in your owner's manual. If not, the ever-popular Google search should supply the answer, if not directly, then through a question asked on a bike forum featuring your make.

Alternator output varies widely among motorcycles, and is dependent upon the intended use of the bike. For example, the alternator output of a 2003 Honda Gold Wing is well over 1,000 watts, whereas a 2002 Honda Shadow puts out 329 of them. Honda knows that a Gold Wing rider will probably load up with power-sapping electrical devices, whereas the Shadow rider not so much.

Now that you know the maximum output of your alternator, the next step is to calculate your operating load. By the way, when you find that alternator output number you'll see that it will read, for example, 675 watts @ 4,000 rpm. What that means is that your motor must be running at a minimum of 4,000 rpm to achieve a maximum output of 675 watts. At idle, or any rpm other than 4,000, the power output would be less.

To calculate operating load you need to add up the power required by all the non-accessory items requiring electrical power. Some of the items are easy. For example, the headlight bulbs; their power requirement will be stamped somewhere on the bulbs, or in your owner's manual. Other items can be time-consuming and a bit tricky. For instance, trying to locate the power required by your fuel injection system can get a little more complicated. You'll probably have to have access to a shop service manual, or the help of a cooperating dealer. Interestingly, the increasing use of original equipment LED lighting on motorcycles has made more power available for accessories, as the power required for LEDs is very low. For example, a 6-watt LED bulb has about the same light emission as a 35-watt halogen bulb.

Let's take a look at a specific example, the specs for my Triumph Tiger 800:

> The **operating-load** power required by the Tiger's fuel injection system, ECM (Electronic Control Module), stock lighting, and ignition comes in at around 250 watts.

The **accessory load** results from these added items:

Auxiliary lights (2)

	24 watts each	=	48
Heated jacket liner			105
Heated gloves	14 watts each	=	28
GPS		=	5

At maximum (high beam, max heat), these items are drawing a total of 186 watts of power.

The maximum output of the Triumph's alternator is 675 watts*. Subtracting the operating load of 250 and the accessory load of 186 watts from that total leaves me with an excess of 239 watts, meaning that I could hook up several other power-sapping devices.

* My owner's manual does not specify alternator output in watts, so I went to the Web and, after a bit of searching, found lots of conflicting information. One site said that the output is 675 watts, another said 700, and that was just two of the numbers I discovered. OK, I thought, let's go about this mathematically; applying Ohm's law shows an output of 523 watts — more than 150 watts *less* than the lowest number (675 watts) that my research found. I've attempted to get clarification from Triumph North America, and the Triumph HQ in England. No luck so far. Using that 523 watt output calculation, I subtract the operating power draw (250 watts) and accessory power draw (186 watts), and I end up with 86 watts of excess available power.

15.

*"It's not that I'm afraid to die, I just don't
want to be there when it happens."*
Woody Allen

Your Mobile Medicine Cabinet

One of the many things that differentiate us old ones from the young ones is the content of our medicine cabinets. Think back to your 20's and your go-to medicine was likely a hangover cure. Today? Well… it's not unusual for that cabinet to contain meds for high blood pressure, acid-reflux problems, high cholesterol, inhalers, ibuprofen, various balms for pain, eye drops, nose drops, and ear drops. And that's just the generic stuff. When you add in the medications you need for specific problems such as diabetes, well, the list of concoctions you need to stay upright and breathing can get very long indeed. Which means when it comes to distance riding and road trips, you need to make some decisions regarding just what to pack.

Let's see if I can simplify this a bit. To start with, there are three categories of medical items that we need to carry. I refer to them as our E-Packs:

1) Emergency Pack
2) Essentials Pack
3) Episode Pack

These packs should be carried separately and packed on our motorcycle as noted below. As with packing anything on a motorcycle, there are some compromises required, so I'm keeping this very basic.

Emergency Pack

There are two critical emergency conditions that you should be prepared for: suffocation and bleeding. If either of these is left unchecked, death is the next step. You need four items to handle these situations, which can be used to save your own life or that of another.

The first item is an **emergency breathing mask**. This is a simple plastic sheet with a one-way valve that protects you from the exchange of bodily fluids if mouth-to-mouth resuscitation is necessary. You place the sheet over the victim's face, centering the valve in their mouth, and force air into them. You should familiarize yourself with the mask's included instructions before you might need it, as every second counts.

The next item you'll need is a **compression bandage**. In a pinch this would be something like an Ace bandage compressing gauze against an open wound. Much more effective is a bandage specifically made for the purpose such as the First Care Products emergency bandage. These are inexpensive and are designed to staunch the flow of blood. Again, familiarize yourself with its use before needing it in an emergency.

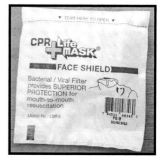

Emergency breathing mask

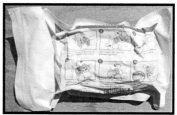

Compression bandage

Serious injury is usually accompanied by circulatory shock wherein the victim's blood pressure can drop to dangerously low levels, depriving the arms and legs of warmth. This can cause uncontrollable shivering that can make the already serious problem even more so. To prevent shock from happening make sure you pack a **space blanket** as part of your Emergency Pack. Also known as a solar blanket this thin sheet of tough, reflective polyester film (generally Mylar) can keep up to 98 percent of a body's heat from escaping. In addition, it is waterproof and can serve as an impromptu shelter and help you stave off *hypothermia*. I don't travel without them, and have found the need for it on a couple of occasions when the night temperature has dropped to an unexpected low while camping.

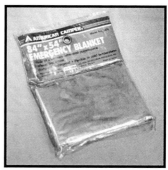

Mylar blanket

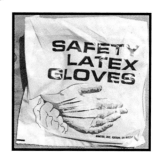

Latex gloves

The fourth item is a pair of **thin rubber gloves**. Anytime blood or fluids are present it's a good idea to have a glove barrier between you and the victim. These four items take up very little space, but having them can make the difference between life and death.

Essentials Pack

Your Essentials Pack should contain your prescribed medications and those over-the-counter meds that you need on a regular basis, such as

---

and this... Warm Hack

If you fit the target age for this book (50-plus), think back to what riders wore to keep warm during your early years of riding. The super-synthetics that we take for granted today, such as Gore-Tex, were still to be developed, so riding gear was heavy on leather, wool, waxed cotton, flannel and denim (the rich guys usually had a silk scarf). Generally, this stuff worked well, but you had to seriously layer it on in really cold weather. Plus, when you did reach a point where you were warm enough, you ended up looking a bit like the Pillsbury doughboy.

Storage was limited on the early motorcycles so a rider usually wore everything they thought they'd need. If you guessed wrong, and the weather turned ugly cold, things could get very uncomfortable, very quickly. If you needed to keep riding, you had to do something to ease the cold. That "something" was a newspaper. (You remember those, right? A multi-layered wood pulp-based, large rectangular thing with lots of words in it.)

What you did was shake the paper to loosen each page, and then stuff it inside your first layer, against your chest. Your body heat (98.6 degrees) would warm up the air held between each page, providing layers of insulation. In extreme cases, you could also line your sleeves with newspaper. This hack worked surprisingly well, unless you got the paper wet. It would then work in reverse, sucking the heat from your body, not to mention the reverse type printed on your chest. The only problem with using this hack today is finding a newspaper.

---

antacid, sunscreen, and bug spray. This is the kit of drugs that probably didn't exist in your world when you began your riding career. Given that these medications are now essential to your health it is important that you pack them carefully in a waterproof container, and pack them somewhere readily accessible. I carry my Essentials Pack in my tank bag as there is usually something in there that I need daily.

If you are on an extended trip it's a good idea to take along your most critical prescriptions. By this, I mean not just the drugs, but also the written prescriptions themselves. Having your written prescriptions with you eliminates any possibility that the legality of your pharmaceutical goody-bag may be questioned. It also makes it significantly easier for you to get a prescription replaced, should you need to do so in a pinch.

Episode Pack

The most important items in this pack are for DAVE, if it comes to visit. That would be diarrhea and vomiting episodes. These are particularly unpleasant conditions at any time, but think about how especially bad it can be while riding a motorcycle.

For most people the go-to over the counter drug for these bits of unpleasantness is Pepto-Bismol, either in liquid or tablet form. In general this pink magic elixir will help with bouts of diarrhea, heartburn, indigestion and upset stomach. Take warning, though: despite it being a non-prescription drug Pepto-Bismol can negatively interact with some other medications, so check with your doctor to confirm compatibility with other medication that you are using.

Your Episode Pack and your Emergency Pack can be stored together in the same place. While you don't need to carry these E-Packs in your tank bag (hopefully you won't need to use them!), it is wise to pack these in a place where you can find them. If possible, always carry them in the same spot in the bottom of the same saddlebag. Remember, if you do find yourself in an emergency situation every second counts.

and this... DAVE

Generally a healthy person won't have to experience DAVE here in the U.S., as our water and food quality is good. However, if you diverge too much from your normal diet, drink too much, or drink water from a questionable source, you and DAVE just might have to share some time together.

The best defense against diarrhea and vomiting should start before the symptoms occur. The most obvious step is to practice good hygiene and, most certainly, this means washing your hands after using the restroom and before eating. This is particularly important when on the road as your system often has to deal with bacteria and viruses that aren't found around your normal environment. Soap and water is the preferred cleansing method, but a bottle of hand sanitizer that contains a minimum of 60% alcohol will work when soap and water are not available. Tests have shown that hand sanitizing liquid is no more effective at sanitizing than a good hand-washing and should only be used if soap and water are not available.

There is increasing concern about the various chemicals used in hand sanitizers. Primary amongst them is the fact that the alcohol can enter the bloodstream through skin absorption and inhalation. Additionally, *triclosan*, a chemical in many of these products, is suspected of adversely effecting heart and skeletal muscles, and is currently under review by the FDA. Because of this, my preferred sanitizer is Purell Advanced, as it does not contain triclosan.

Another way to avoid sickness is to pay attention to what you're eating. Undercooked meat is a major cause of intestinal problems. When in doubt, ask for that juicy hamburger to be cooked well done. Fresh fruit and vegetables are some of the best things you can eat for overall body health, but be careful with them. Ideally, fruit that you peel, such as bananas, are the safest but you should always wash, or peel, any other fruit that you might buy at a roadside stand. The same with vegetables; raw carrots are a great, healthy snack, but unless you can wash them, stick with the well-cooked variety.

When I was a boy, the Dead Sea was only sick.
George Burns

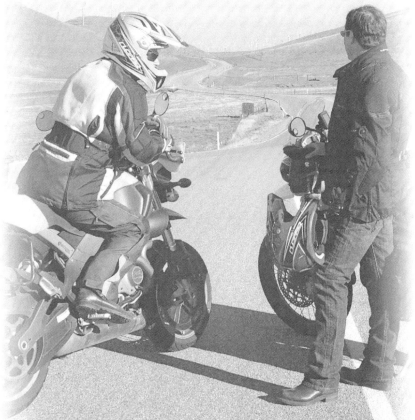

in other words

words

Phil Ammendolia
Wendy Perry

Phil Ammendolia, 56

It's a sport and hobby I share with my family

Some of the youngest people I know are motorcyclists over the age of 50. My life of riding started like many; bumming a ride on my friend's Taco minibike when I was about 9 years old. I was hooked immediately, and have been fortunate to turn my passion into my career. That has given me many decades to observe the changes in those around me and has allowed me to pick the path that I will follow.

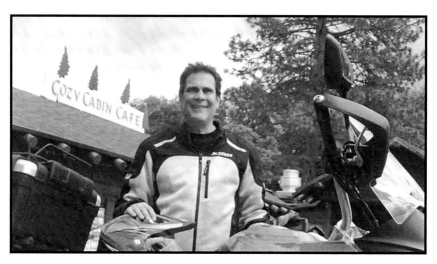

Like many, when I was a kid, I thought I was going to be a rocket and make my living riding a motorcycle. I was wrong. But the cool thing about motorcycles is that despite not being a contender to a world title, I still get to participate. "Racing" is something I can do almost any week-end I choose. There are a lot of events that are titled a "race," where there are a lot of other old kids like me that are about the same skill level and can offer a real battle, but know they need to show up for work on Monday, just like I do. Racing, even at my level, has given me a goal in life. Since I was a teenager, I've raced in every decade. My plan is to keep that going, even if it's just a local "run what you brung," through my 70's. Then I want to ride my dual-sport bike to the track and watch from the pit wall when I'm 80.

One of the observations made through the years is that, though we may all limp a little more, or get up a little more slowly, motorcyclists tend to be younger in their mindset than most of the other people I've known. There's camaraderie; there's a spirit of adventure; and there's a sense of accomplishment after a hard ride that I just haven't found elsewhere. That's most apparent when I consider the friendships I've developed through the years, some of which have lasted well over 40 years. There are few places in the U.S. that I travel that there isn't some-one nearby that I can call a friend. And most importantly, as a group, I believe we tend to enjoy life at a level that many others never experience. It's a sport and

I thought I was going to be a rocket and make my living riding a motorcycle.

hobby I share with my family and I believe it's made my relationships better. We certainly share a life full of great memories.

It doesn't matter if it's a run to the store for a carton of milk, or a weeklong, 400-mile-a-day journey. For me, life is better when viewed from the seat of a motorcycle.

Wendy Perry, 64

You Just Can't Keep a Great Woman Down

At the age of 34 I was a late bloomer to motorcycling, but made up for lost time after my initial motorcycle training course, trading up in rapid succession through two small Japanese bikes and a 1986 883 Sportster, until I found the bike of my dreams in the 1988 Springer Soft-tail. That bike and I laid down 96,000 miles in the eight years we rode together, and in 1997 I moved on to yet another Springer Softtail. Due to my smallish stature nothing else on the market at the time fit so well.

In January of 2000, my 50th year, I tore my rotator cuff in a non-motorcycle related incident and had surgery to repair it, all the while anticipating getting back on

I can still racket around town on my ever so bitchin' Springer

the bike as soon as possible. Women, we all are reminded regularly, are woefully lacking in upper body strength, so to this day I faithfully carry out the exercise routine that I learned in physical therapy.

In 2005, I was diagnosed with a back situation that required surgery. The physical beating inflicted while enjoying the first twenty-one years of my motorcycling career just managed to contribute to the pre-existing damage I had sustained with my many years of long-distance running. And all the time I was just trying to stay healthy. At that point it was necessary to acknowledge that the Springer was a little rough on my 55-year-old body. I was frequently reminded of this when, at the end of a riding day, while my traveling buddies were heading to the bar, I was crawling into bed, exhausted and aching. I found that the Deluxe Soft-

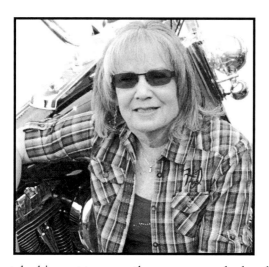

tail new to the market rode incredibly smoothly, and with some slight modifications to the exhaust so that I could add a set of Heritage Softtail saddlebags, I was set with my new touring bike.

Now, even after my 2012 hip replacement, I can still racket around town on my ever so bitchin' Springer, and even take him out to carve the canyons, as he handles so much quicker than the Deluxe, but when the going calls for long distance it is great to have the smooth cruiser for the sake of comfort and stamina.

Last September I went to the doctor for a cortisone shot in my shoulder prior to riding to New Mexico. I thought I was just dealing with some arthritis, but, due to my symptoms and after an annoying test that he put me through, I was diagnosed with carpal tunnel issues. I had my right hand operated on in March and we'll do the left in April. It will be so nice to have feeling in my 64-year-old hands and arms.

During that diagnostic visit, learning that I would be riding through mountains, the doctor asked me if I ever had any problems breathing at altitudes. I told him I used to have a hard time with my older bike, but that my new one was fuel-injected. He gave me the strangest look.

16.

*A very old rider tells his friend, "I think my new
GPS unit is defective."
"What makes you think so?" asks the friend.
"Well, I used it for the first time this morning, and the first
thing it said was, 'Ride 200 feet and let me off!'"*

Arké

Getting Found

Getting lost while on a motorcycle trip used to be my norm.
Whether it was from inexperience, poor planning, or an attack
of the stupids, I could count on finding myself somewhere I didn't figure
to be — and not knowing just where that was — at least once on any
lengthy trip. Generally I could count on my good sense of direction to
get me out of those predicaments, and eventually I learned that a bit
more time spent planning the trip, and a decent set of maps, could eliminate those, "I'm not lost, I just don't know where I am" moments. This is
true of most older, more experienced riders: been there, done that, asked
for directions, it all worked out. Today, given the GPS technology that is
readily available, if you find yourself truly lost it means that either you're
a technophobe or you really want to be lost. Eventually most riders get
the "getting lost" problem under control, but what about the "getting
found" part? What if you take a wrong turn off a cliff and need emergency rescue workers to locate you?

There are really no good excuses for getting lost, staying lost, or
not getting found. It is simply a
matter of taking a few preventive
steps. While I love the idea of just
striking out and letting impulse
decide my direction, this only
really works if I'm not due back in the near future and there's no one at
home concerned about me. As neither of those conditions mirror my life,
before I leave the house on a long ride, I always take a few steps to make

*There are really no good excuses
for getting lost, staying lost, or
not getting found.*

199

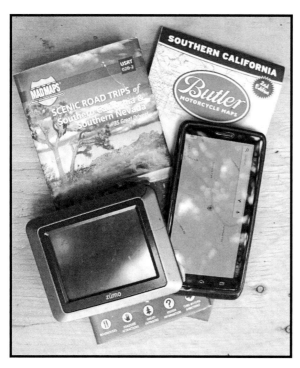

sure I know where I'm going and how I may be found should the need arise.

The first step is to leave a clear map at home showing my intended route. Secondly, I tell my wife when I'll be checking in with her; generally, this is every morning, but she also knows that if I miss a call-in, not to worry.

The third step is to decide what I will take with me in my lost/found kit. This can vary depending upon trip duration, but the one constant is always my cellphone. More specifically, a smartphone. I've had a few riders tell me that their cellphone is the first thing they leave behind when taking off on their motorcycle. This romantic notion ("...leaving it all behind") works right up until you really need that phone. And by the way.... Tried to find a pay phone lately?

Smartphones are marvels of technology that can provide a rider with far more than just the ability to call home. They can be critical in determining where you're at, not only for your sake, but also for someone who might be looking for you. To begin with, most all smartphones are equipped with a global positioning system (GPS) receiver. This "GPS chip" can tell you within a few feet exactly where you are, and pinpoint your location on a map. This is a pretty good way to get un-lost.

Equally important is that your smartphone or your standard cellphone can also get you found. If you are able to reach a 911 connection (in other words, if you have phone service) but are unable to talk, you can be located by the data gathered from the cell towers in your vicinity. And here's another bit of trickery. If you are using a smartphone and have reached a 911 operator, they can actually turn your smartphone's GPS function on if you are unable to do so. What all this means is that, turned on or not, your phone (smart, or not) can get you found.

And another getting found angle to consider. If the folks back home haven't heard from you and believe that something bad has happened, they should, of course, contact the police. The police can then get in touch with your cellphone service provider (Verizon, Sprint, AT&T, et al.). Then... here's where it gets interesting. As long as your phone is on, the cellphone network is continually scanning your phone to make sure that the nearest tower is available to you when you need to make a call. As you travel, this contact moves from tower to tower. What this scanning allows the service provider to do is analyze the signal strength from three different towers nearest you then, using a triangulation formula, they can determine your approximate whereabouts. Remember, though, your phone has to be on for this to work.

It's important to understand that the GPS chip works differently from the phone function. When you initiate or receive a call, your phone is working with nearby cellphone tower sites. As your phone requires a clear "line of sight" to a cell tower, you will find very spotty or nonexistent phone service in heavily wooded or remote areas. The GPS function, however, works with a network of orbiting satellites totally independent of cellphone service. What this means is that as long as you can power

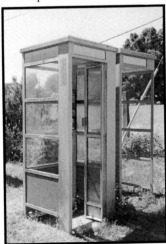

up your phone (and get out from under the trees), you will be able to determine your location, even though you cannot call out.

And that is how you can be found.

(Still want to leave that phone home?)

Here SPOT!

The problem with writing about new technology is the rapidity with which it can become old technology. This is particularly true when it comes to electronic devices. However, despite this fact there is a bit of newish tech that I think you need to know

Not a "smartphone," but an answer to a trivia question.

about as it could save your hide in certain situations: personal tracking devices. In what follows I mention the SPOT brand because it is the one I've been using for several years. There are, however, numerous other manufacturers such as Bushnell, Celestron and DeLorme that provide the same services.

SPOT is its name, and finding you is its game. This is a GPS tracking device —or Satellite GPS Messenger as called by the company— that you carry with you. When activated, it emits a signal every 10 minutes. Within

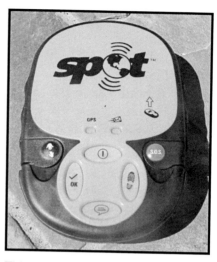

This is my SPOT, about 2.5-in. x 4-in. The newest ones are a bit smaller.

about 15 minutes, this signal appears as a plot on a Google map (if you've signed up for that option). The fun part here is that your envious (and nosy) friends can now track your trip, mile by mile. Additionally, if they switch to Google's "Earth" view they can see the actual terrain you're traversing, though not, obviously, at the time you are there.

Ultimately, SPOT's primary purpose is to summon aid in the event that you are injured and cannot ride. By pressing a small button beneath a protective cover a signal is sent to GEOS, an "International Emergency Response Coordination Center." In turn, GEOS notifies those you've listed as contacts and appropriate rescue organizations. In addition to the initial cost, an annual service charge is required. Just how much this is depends upon the various services that you need, or want. In my case it costs me about one hundred bucks a year. I consider that cheap given the piece of mind that it offers both my wife and myself. If you've a spouse and or others that follow you it's helpful to give them a heads up as to how to interpret the computer tracking. In particular I've told her not to be concerned if she sees that I'm stopped for an extended period of time in the middle of nowhere because either a) I'm taking pictures, b) answering nature's call or, b) I'm taking a nap.

Ideally SPOT should be mounted somewhere on your body where it won't be knocked off in the event of a crash; the chest area works well, but definitely not on your helmet. Also, place it externally, not in a pocket, so that the built-in antenna (similar to a cellphone) can easily access a satellite.

...more on GPS

The Global Positioning System is probably one of the best deals our government has ever given us, and yet most don't really understand it, or take advantage of all it has to offer. The origins of GPS go back to the late 1950's where it evolved into, initially, a navigation and weapon's targeting system for the U.S. military. In turn this became NAVSTAR (Navigation Satellite Timing and Ranging), the official name of our GPS system. NAVSTAR is controlled by the U.S. Department of Defense. The system consists of 24 satellites orbiting at a 12,000-mile altitude, with each circling the earth twice in a 24-hour period. Each one of these satellites continuously emits a radio signal and at any given time four of these satellites can be electronically "visible" (via that radio signal) to that GPS receiver clamped to your handlebars. I say, "can be" because the radio signal must have a clear line of sight to and from your GPS unit. Heavy tree covering, tunnels and similar obstructions will interrupt the signal.

To fully understand how GPS works, we'd have to get deep into Doppler shift, 3D trilateration and math formulas that would put all of us to sleep and confuse the hell out of me. I'm not going there because while that might be fun information for some, it is not really necessary for our purposes. It suffices to know that your GPS receiver knows precisely where each of those four "visible" satellites is located. With the information contained in the signals from the satellites —and the map program stored within the receiver— your GPS unit can display your location as close as within 10 feet of your actual location. Interestingly, the military and civilian GPS signals were at one time intentionally different, with the military having access to the more accurate signal. Today, the signals are the same. However, the military is able to correct for signal degradation as it traverses the ionosphere. This gives it a higher degree of accuracy and allows the targeting of the bad guys in hidden-away bunkers.

"So what?" you might ask. Well, here's what. Those radio signals from the incredibly expensive NAVSTAR system, and your inexpensive GPS unit can tell you, among other things:
- where you are located
- how fast you are traveling
- your average speed, overall
- your moving average speed
- trip time, overall
- moving time
- estimated arrival time
- moving direction
- how fast you are traveling
- your altitude

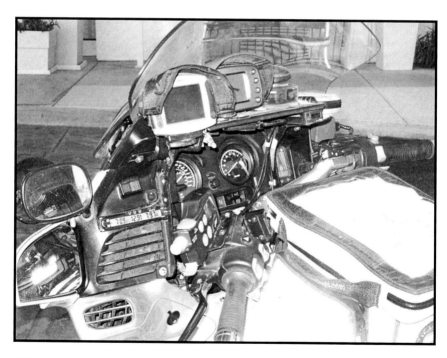

I like my electro-doo-dads as well as the next guy, but I do have a limit. This rider has managed to pack on two GPS systems, two satellite trackers, numerous lights, weather monitors and a comm system. And then there's those four rearview mirrors. It would be interesting to know just how much power all these draw.

I've used a GPS unit on my motorcycle for several years and have come to depend upon it for many reasons, but not necessarily the most obvious one; knowing where I'm located. I've had non-GPS users ask me, "Why do I need to spend money for something to tell me where I am, as I always know that?" Good question, and were that the only reason to own one, I'd say pass on it. However, for me that is almost the least of reasons why I use one. Its two most useful functions are the ability to direct me to a new location via turn-by-turn instructions, and the continual updating of my estimated arrival time at the destination I've entered. I also like the average speed readouts as they keep me on schedule when I have to be somewhere at a specific time. Additionally, I've come to depend upon the speed readout as most experts state it to be more accurate than a speedometer. Many also claim that speedometers are calibrated a bit "optimistically" so as to give drivers a margin for speed error. The unit I currently have (Garmin Zumo 220) also has a handy nanny feature in that it can tell me when I'm getting low on gas and highlight nearby gas stations. This is particularly important in the more remote areas.

As much as I like using GPS, it does not completely replace the paper map for me. The screen is just too small for trip planning, and I like being able to see the big picture. Paper is also handy for trip notes, and paper maps offer more information as regards road type and quality. Oddly, I've found more errors with GPS maps than with the paper versions. I say "oddly" because GPS data is updated on a regular basis, whereas paper maps are often years old.

17.

The word adventure has gotten overused. For me, when everything goes wrong, that's when adventure starts.

Yvon Chouinard

Thoughts on Motorcycle Camping

When I raise the subject of a possible camping trip with older riding friends, most hastily change the subject or look at me as if I'm missing more than a few fries in my Big Meal. Before you run off to the next chapter ...hear me out. Motorcycle camping can add a whole new enjoyable page to your motorcycle resume. And I believe it can help you extend your riding career.

Think back to your trips when you were younger. Hotels and motels were probably your choice for a night's rest. And if you were riding with a group the usual post-dinner meeting place was probably the

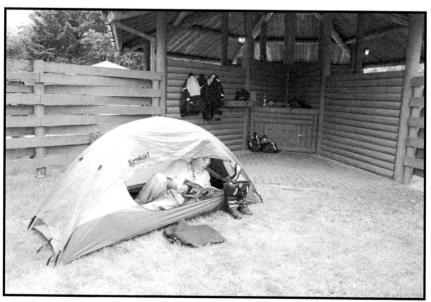

One of the nicest KOA (Kampgrounds of America) campgrounds is in Astoria, Oregon. You have your own lockable corral, secure storage, general store, patio, a nice lawn, and peace and quiet.

...and one of the worst:

KOA Las Vegas. A patch of burnt grass in a noisy parking lot full of noisy kids, next to a noisy casino.

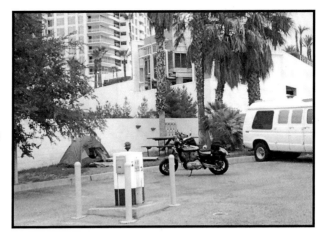

resident bar or nearby watering hole. I've had many memorable nights — and a few I can't remember— doing just that. Attendant to some of those were mornings that arrived too early and much too loudly. As I've never been a heavy drinker it didn't take much to put me under the table. As I grew older I tapered off on the revelry, started going to bed earlier and found —Surprise! Surprise!— I was enjoying the mornings much more, not to mention getting earlier starts. This change in lifestyle is common, but as I was, and am, usually older than those with whom I've ridden, I often found myself the first to back away from the party scene.

While no one would mistake me for Mark Trail (you gotta be old to know who he is) I've always enjoyed camping, so when I began to combine this with my riding I discovered the two activities matched perfectly.

I like motorcycle camping for several reasons. Not only because it is a change from my normal home-based routine, but also because it involves a completely different dynamic from the motel-to-motel sprint. Additionally, while it may be illusionary, I like the idea that I have to be a bit more self-sufficient when camping. And as a huge benefit from this, I find that I sleep better and in general feel better than when I motel it.

It is not my intent to get too deep into motorcycle camping equipment —that's a large book in itself. I do, though, want to address the primary reason that riders have given me for not camping: discomfort.

When I talk about motorcycle camping with riders one thing is continually mentioned: comfort, or rather, lack of it. And that used to be the norm. If you were an occasional camper you could count on sleeping fitfully, being cold, and eating badly. Those who camped regularly knew how to solve these problems, or learned to tolerate them. Every time I see an old picture with a bedroll tied to the bars I can't help but think of what an uncomfortable night that rider must have spent. Today, if you're cold, uncomfortable, or can't sleep while you're camping, you've no one to blame but yourself as camping technology has solved all the discomfort problems.

Comfortable Camping

I don't get along with cold at all. Those who know me sometimes shake their heads at my intolerance to temperature drops, and my wife and I are continually at odds regarding thermostats and open doors and windows. Couple this with the fact that old age and various past injuries do not tolerate sleeping on the hard ground, and you might think me the last to camp out. More correctly, I'm the first to suggest it. And this is because I've solved the sleeping/cold puzzle.

Sleeping Warm and Comfy

A good night's sleep requires only that you be comfortable, and there are two components to that; 1) how your sleeping bag fits and, 2) how warm and dry you remain.

Bag Fit

There are two basic configurations of sleeping bags: square and mummy. A square bag is, essentially, insulating material and a cover, folded in half, with a zipper down one side. A mummy bag is narrower, somewhat cone-shaped, has an integral hood, and a zipper which only partially extends down one side.

Bag Insulation

Sleeping bag insulating material is either synthetic or down.   Synthetic-filled bags are less expensive and easier to maintain. However, they do not insulate as well as down-filled bags, are heavier, and do not compress to as small a package. There are several

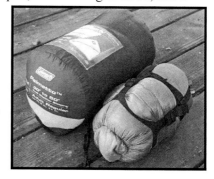

The down bag on the right packs significantly smaller than the synthetic bag, but for sleeping comfort I prefer the synthetic.

different synthetics available, including Polargard, Quallofil, and Hollofil, with each having different use characteristics. Before you buy a synthetic bag it would pay to do a bit of research regarding each synthetic filling. Down-filled bags offer superior warmth, are lighter, and pack very small. They are, however, more expensive and fail to work at all if they get wet. By the way, "down" is the layer of feathers of a bird that are just beneath the outer feathers. Generally, goose down is used.

After having used several variations of sleeping bags over the years, my preference is a synthetic-filled square bag. I don't like how a mummy bag restricts movement, and that insulation's problem with water. A square bag is generally thought of as a casual-use item, as it does not trap heat as does a mummy bag. I solve this problem by always packing winter-weight long underwear. Were I a backpacker, I'd go the mummy/down route, but as weight and size are not that big an issue on a motorcycle, I'll stick with the more comfy square bag.

Obviously, camping with just a sleeping bag is not sufficient to meet the comfortable/warm/dry requirements. You also need a good tent and a decent insulating mattress, but without that correct sleeping bag you might as well stay home because your camping experience will not be all that pleasant.

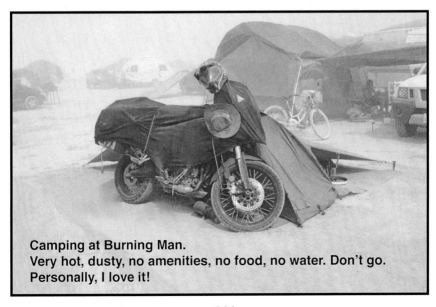

Camping at Burning Man.
Very hot, dusty, no amenities, no food, no water. Don't go.
Personally, I love it!

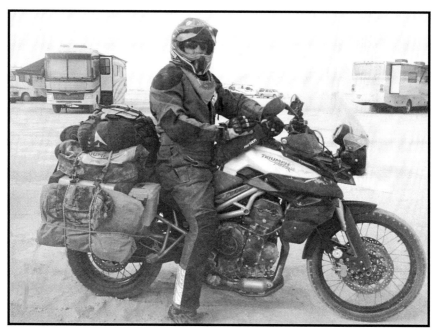

Everything I need for six days of camping, except water.

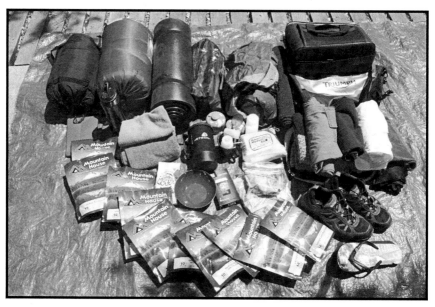

A typical load for a five day camping trip.

18.

Life is not meant to be all homogenized and pasteurized.
Gotta live, love and laugh. And ride too.

Brian Ratliff

To Ride, or Not

Not everyone should ride a motorcycle, regardless of his or her age. To safely and competently ride takes a level of concentration and coordination that not everyone has. Many of the necessary skills can be learned, but there are some people that never feel comfortable riding and as such, they shouldn't. Ultimately, this decision has to come from the potential rider as the purchase of a motorcycle only requires money, and passing the licensing procedure in this country needs little more than a pulse. This to-ride-or-not decision has to be made at two points in a rider's history: in the beginning, and at the end.

In the Beginning...

The pattern is a common one. A 50-ish man has jumped through all the job hoops, just about has the kids out of the house, and has a few bucks in the bank. He's always wanted a motorcycle. The dealer and the state are happy to oblige. More often this motorcycle dream has been centered around a Harley-Davidson. And this is understandable as The Motor Company makes beautiful machines, steeped in history, and wrapped in the flag. They are also large, heavy machines that may not be the best motorcycles on which to begin a late-starting riding career. If the above comes close to describing you then you need to access the wisdom you gained over the years and think hard about your decision.

First, the physical end of things. Are you reasonably coordinated? If your shins are dented from running into things, your hands laced with scars from inept tool use, and your car wears a patina of dents, I'd think twice about getting on a motorcycle. Seriously. A pattern of those things indicates a condition that might be laughable to those around you (you're not ill, just clumsy), but is anything but funny on a motorcycle. Consider this: the situation that produced any one of those dents in your car would have far more serious consequences on a motorcycle. And what about your balance? If you've any issues with balance I strongly suggest that a motorcycle is not for you.

Your first step should be a consultation with your doctor. Tell him what your plans are and listen to his opinion. Know this though: the medical profession is not necessarily the biggest booster of riding. So you'll have to get him past the lecture phase before he can tell you if he sees any condition with you that would preclude riding.

What about your head? Not its shape, but what's in it. Successful riding requires that you be assertive. You need to be able to make quick decisions and decisively act on them. If by nature you are a very deliberate sort that likes to take your time to suss out all the options and ramifications of your actions, well, you're probably an excellent financial planner but not necessarily a good motorcycle rider. Situations can develop very quickly on a motorcycle and you need to be able to react just as quickly, if not quicker.

Many riders confuse assertive riding with aggressive riding.

Many riders — particularly young ones — confuse assertive riding with aggressive riding. The differences can be subtle, but their effects can often mean the difference between a motorcycle ride or an ambulance ride. Four-way intersections often reveal the difference between riding aggression and assertion. The aggressive rider challenges the traffic; "Hey, it's my turn and I'm taking it." The assertive rider recognizes that a car coming from the left does not have the right of away, but that it's going to cross his path regardless.

In many ways a motorcycle rider is analogous to a pedestrian. They may have the legal right of way, but the laws of physics always trump the laws of the state. You don't want your tombstone to read, "But I had the right of way!"

The decision to ride or not must also include your family. Riding a motorcycle can be a high-risk activity with your physical well-being, and possibly your life, at stake. To ride without the support of those who care for and depend upon you is a selfish act. The good news in this is that you can significantly reduce your risk by using your head not only as a helmet holder, but also for logical thinking.

...And at the End

Regardless of our age and current physical/mental condition, there will come a day when we have to hang our helmets up for the last time. While the overriding goal of this book is to extend our riding days, we know that day we hang it up will be sooner, rather than later. For those of us who have ridden for decades, that will be very difficult to do.

The decision to not ride should be a personal one, and not one forced upon us by doctors or our families. I say this for two reasons. First, because making the decision yourself is part of being a responsible, competent rider and, second, because we should be the first to know when our skills

Everyone has an occasional bad riding day. It wasn't necessarily catastrophic, just a day where things were just a bit... off.

have slipped to the point where we're a danger to ourselves or others.

Everyone has an occasional bad riding day. It wasn't necessarily catastrophic, just a day where things were just a bit... off. Maybe our mind was wandering, or we were not feeling well. Generally we shake it off, or turn back to the garage, knowing that the next ride will be better. And it always has been. But at some point it won't be. The problem arises when those bad riding days start to string together, where every ride is just a bit off. There might be too many near misses, or stupid mistakes like neglecting to downshift when coming to a stop, or forgetting to raise the side stand.

There can be several reasons for this with illness and fatigue at the top of the list, as these conditions tend to fog our thinking and slow our reactions. As this book has shown, we can do something about these conditions to a certain extent. But, inevitably — despite our efforts —our skills will degrade to the point where it becomes recklessly stupid to continue riding.

Red Flags Waving

There are numerous red flags that warn of the end of our riding career. That we might have experienced some of these is not a reason to panic, but if a pattern of miscues has developed it's probably time to rethink our riding.

Falling down or crashing

This doesn't need a lot of explanation. If you're doing this with any regularity, you should not be riding with any regularity —or at all.

Near misses

If every ride features one of those "Whoa!" moments where you just narrowly avoid an accident, this is a big red flag.

Surprise! Surprise!

If you often find yourself saying, "Where'd he come from?" it indicates that you're not focusing on riding, and that your situational awareness skills may no longer be as sharp as necessary.

And then there are these...

Are you getting honked at a lot?
Are you riding significantly below the speed limit?
Are you having difficulty reading street signs or
    discerning the colors on stoplights?
Are those close to you dropping hints about
    retiring from the saddle?

I mentioned above that the decision to hang up the helmet should be a personal one, but a part of the decision can come from those close to us, and our riding partners. Ask them how they feel about your riding. You might get your feelings hurt, but it also might save your life.

Do not go gentle into that good night,
Old age should burn and rave at close of day;
Rage, rage against the dying of the light.

in other words

words

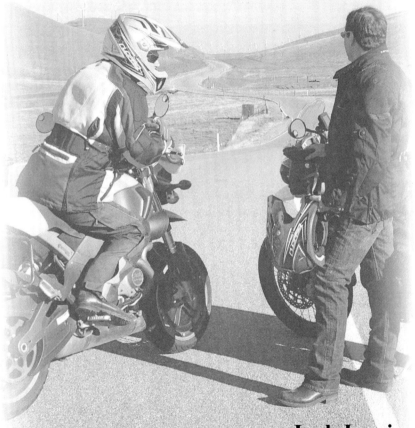

Jack Lewis

Jack Lewis, 51

A Golden Age Rage

We live in a fallen world. No points to file, jets to swap, kick start-ers, or petcocks. Engines are tuned with laptops (or maybe your phone); suspension is adjusted from your handlebar. Riders hardly even wave at each other now. When you see a brother pulled over by the roadside, he's probably just taking a call.

From his boyfriend.

Where have all the real riders gone, those men of iron on steel steeds who used to be us? They're not lurking around dealerships, hop-ing to eavesdrop on the arcana of desmodromic valves; bike deals are mediated through Costco these days, like farmed salmon and toilet paper. They're not pre-mixing premium fuel for their dirt bikes; two-smokes have gone the way of Tin Lizzie and the party line – but you remember when they were new and revolutionary, don't you? When it took a ba-dass to pull the trigger on a TZ750, and the rest of we mortals sputtered through town on RD350s and pretended we were King Kenny for a day.

Every piece of riding can be better than it ever was, if you make it that way. Run your bike to the store, take a course, blast a track day, ride the Alps, do doughnuts in the dirt with your grandkids.

We bitch because we can't see into the black boxes without a com-puter, and delude ourselves that familiar old tech made us better, because in some mysterious way it "built character." Which makes as much sense as B&W film photojournalists griping about cellphone cameras that make better pictures than their top-shelf Nikons did, back in the day when auto-winders were rare, expensive, professional tools and every lensman had to mind his own f-stops, speed, and focus. Are the pictures better when they're harder to obtain? Or does technology exist – and advance – for a reason?

Unless you once ground your own pigments from bone char, raw umber and lapis lazuli to daub on cave walls with a stick, you've no business carping about DSLRs steepening the learning curve of represen-tational imagery and if the last bike you bought isn't kick-start only, it's time to face the techno-beat music, Pops.

Also, you're either not 25 or you're reading the wrong book, so you know damn well that old trick knee of yours probably only has one brutal kickback in it before your next surgery and an eight-month rehab. Ain't nobody got time fo' dat!

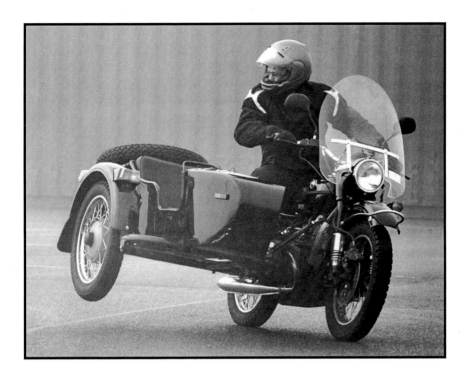

Here's the good news: that vividly tasteless, punk equipment you see whining up and down the street where you live is orders of magnitude better than anything you could buy when you were young enough to want – nay, need – the best. Today's average middleweight is faster and handles better than the million-dollar race bikes Yamaha crushed after each season during the fabulous Seventies.

Instead of griping that 200-hp superbikes weren't around when you were young (instead of being wasted on today's feckless but speedy youth), celebrate the fact that you can afford to ride what you want now. Enjoy riding motorcycles that start every time, on the button, without having to tickle the carbs. Be honest: not only do you not miss the petcock ritual, you're gonna forget it half the time, anyway. If you don't believe that, look down and check your fly.

Street tires that actually stick, rain or shine, and hold pressure for weeks – betcha never saw that coming. Gear that protects you in reasonable comfort, GPS navigation and big, bright headlights – of course you don't need any of that newfangled crap. You're old school, baby, as tough as they come – but don't those heated grips feel nice on a bone-cold day?

The Golden Age of anything is only seen in retrospect, but I encourage you to revel in yours today. Yesterday is for memory and perspective. It's all those things that sucked that make for great stories, and you already have a fund of those. Now that you know what you like, go gitcha some.

Every piece of riding can be better than it ever was, if you make it that way. Run your bike to the store, take a course, blast a track day, ride the Alps, do doughnuts in the dirt with your grandkids. Ride a hog if it feels cool, a super bike if you want to test your reflexes, or a scooter if it makes you grin. Enjoy being called "sir" by the nice young patrolman as he writes you a warning instead of tasing your felonious old butt.

Just remember to pay attention, and wear good gear. You don't want to break a hip.

No, I'm serious about that.

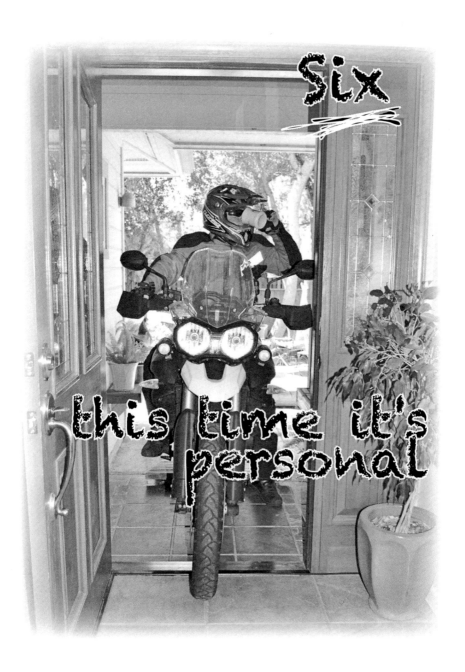

Six

this time it's personal

19.

A Work in Progress

I've offered up a lot of fact and opinion to get to this point, but all of it can be summed up in a couple of paragraphs.

Much of what we consider "normal" in the aging process is really nothing more than laziness on our part. It's a simple process: As we become less active, our bodies deteriorate. In particular, our muscles wither, our bones weaken, and our cardiovascular system becomes a candidate for a plumber's snake. Furthermore, as we put less physical demands on our bodies the need for a healthful, energy-providing diet decreases and we resort to eating "feel good" food that ranks very low on the nutrition scale. All of this can result in a weakened body, a sluggish mind, and the premature retiring of our motorcycle helmets to a dusty corner of our "What Once Was" cabinet.

The good news is that this simple process works both ways. As we become more active, our bodies improve. In particular, we build muscle, strengthen our bones, and help keep our cardiovascular system operating at high efficiency. Furthermore, as we put increased physical demands on our bodies the need for a healthful, energy-providing diet increases and we focus on eating foods from the positive end of that nutrition scale. The result is a stronger body, a sharper mind, and the extension of our riding career well into old age.

As for me...

"If I knew I was going to live this long, I'd have taken better care of myself," is a quote attributed to many different people. While the origin argument might be important to others, the sentiment can't be argued and probably applies to most of us who have reached decades on the far side of 50. I'd like to believe that had I known 30 years ago what I know today (about aging) I would have done some things differently. The reality is it probably would not have made a difference in my behavior.

I know this because I know me; I need goals, incentives, and deadlines. Thirty years ago I was ignorantly happy with both my physical condition and my riding, and paid little thought to living in my 70's. What changed is stated in the very first sentence of this book, "I was noticing that my riding was getting a bit sloppy." That was my incentive to changes some things about my life.

Personally, I'm a work in progress and will be till my last breath. And this is the way it should be as acceptance of the status quo —to my mind— is quite boring, and a shortcut to the endless dirt nap. For the most part I'm satisfied with my progress. My overall physically strength has increased significantly, particularly with my legs. This has resulted in improved riding control and precision. No, this effort hasn't turned me into that two-wheeled hero I never was; it has simply made me a better, more competent rider, and a rider who is better prepared to continue riding despite my age.

Dealing with CTS and STT Arthritis

I'm going to tell you about my aches and pains because both the conditions I mention here are very common to older people, they can seriously impact motorcycle riding, and this information may help make you a better rider. That's why. Now… moving on…

About two-thirds of my way through this book the pain that I'd been experiencing in my dominant left hand advanced from, "that's annoying," to "uh, doctor's appointment." Four doctors, two physical therapists, and one acupuncturist later it was determined that my left hand was suffering from carpal tunnel syndrome (CTS) and STT arthritis. My hand's flexibility was significantly reduced front-to-rear, side-to-side motion was very painful, and my grip strength had fallen from 122 pounds to 99 pounds. Obviously this put a damper on a lot of my strength exercises including push-ups, pull-ups, and anything to do with barbells over my head. Oh, and riding. The pain had reached a level where holding on to the left grip was very difficult. The surgeon diagnosed both the CTS and STT arthritis as "severe," meaning I had to do something about them if I wanted to continue exercising, let alone riding.

The carpal tunnel problem was taken care of by a simple bit of "minimally invasive" surgery. This involved a small half-inch incision, a flexible tube with a camera and a light at the end (endoscope), and a deft surgeon with small tools. Within two days the slight pain and discomfort from this procedure was gone, as was the characteristic numbness in my palm and third and little finger was gone. (Good job, Doc!)

STT (*scaphotrapezotrapezoidal*) arthritis is so named because it affects the scaphoid, trapezium, and trapezoid wrist bones. This is a degenerative type of arthritis that causes the cartilage at the ends of the bone to wear away, allowing the bones themselves to painfully contact each other. The bones in question are adjacent to the thumb. This is a very common form of arthritis.

If I was sedentary and carefully minimized straining my hand, a daily dose of ibuprofen would work to control the pain. In discussing my

The white plastic brace allows me to do *most* exercises, except for anything overhead. Additionally, I wear gloves with with Velcro cuffs which I fit tightly. This wrist support will get me through an exercise session.

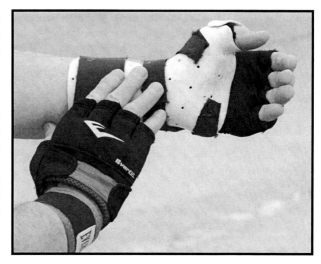

options with the doc I prefaced things by telling him, "I'm not ready to sit on the porch and let life pass by." To his credit he understood and questioned me at length as to how I use my hands. In a nutshell I told him, "I ride a motorcycle. I build things. I like tools. I exercise." He told me that ultimately surgery would probably be necessary, and that this could take several forms but all involve the removal of bones, or bone portions. In the interim he wanted to try a corticosteroid injection in my wrist, a common treatment for joint problems. When I asked him how long I would benefit from this he could not be specific as he'd seen it last "anywhere from a week to more than two years." Sounded like the preferred option to me.